Management of Complex Female Genital Malformations

Management of Complex Female Genital Malformations

Editor

K. Katharina Rall

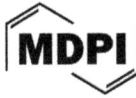

Basel • Beijing • Wuhan • Barcelona • Belgrade • Novi Sad • Cluj • Manchester

Editor
K. Katharina Rall
Department of Women's Health,
Tuebingen University Hospital
Tuebingen, Germany

Editorial Office
MDPI
St. Alban-Anlage 66
4052 Basel, Switzerland

This is a reprint of articles from the Special Issue published online in the open access journal *Journal of Clinical Medicine* (ISSN 2077-0383) (available at: https://www.mdpi.com/journal/jcm/special_issues/Complex_Female_Genital_Malformations).

For citation purposes, cite each article independently as indicated on the article page online and as indicated below:

Lastname, A.A.; Lastname, B.B. Article Title. *Journal Name* **Year**, *Volume Number*, Page Range.

ISBN 978-3-0365-9945-8 (Hbk)
ISBN 978-3-0365-9946-5 (PDF)
doi.org/10.3390/books978-3-0365-9946-5

© 2024 by the authors. Articles in this book are Open Access and distributed under the Creative Commons Attribution (CC BY) license. The book as a whole is distributed by MDPI under the terms and conditions of the Creative Commons Attribution-NonCommercial-NoDerivs (CC BY-NC-ND) license.

Contents

Iori Kisu, Miho Iida, Kanako Nakamura, Kouji Banno, Tetsuro Shiraishi, Asahi Tokuoka, et al.
Laparoscopic Vaginoplasty Procedure Using a Modified Peritoneal Pull-Down Technique with Uterine Strand Incision in Patients with Mayer–Rokitansky–Küster–Hauser Syndrome: Kisu Modification
Reprinted from: *J. Clin. Med.* **2021**, *10*, 5510, doi:10.3390/jcm10235510 1

Katja Wechsung, Louise Marshall, Martina Jürgensen, Uta Neumann and on behalf of the Empower-DSD Study Group
Diagnosis of DSD in Children—Development of New Tools for a Structured Diagnostic and Information Management Program within the Empower-DSD Study
Reprinted from: *J. Clin. Med.* **2022**, *11*, 3859, doi:10.3390/jcm11133859 11

Eva Porsius, Marian Spath, Kirsten Kluivers, Willemijn Klein and Hedi Claahsen-van der Grinten
Primary Amenorrhea with Apparently Absent Uterus: A Report of Three Cases
Reprinted from: *J. Clin. Med.* **2022**, *11*, 4305, doi:10.3390/jcm11154305 25

Lea Tschaidse, Matthias K. Auer, Ilja Dubinski, Christian Lottspeich, Hanna Nowotny, Heinrich Schmidt, et al.
Ectopic Prostate Tissue in the Uterine Cervix of a Female with Non-Classic Congenital Adrenal Hyperplasia—A Case Report
Reprinted from: *J. Clin. Med.* **2022**, *11*, 4307, doi:10.3390/jcm11154307 33

Gina Tonkin-Hill, Chloe Hanna, Roberto Bonelli, Rowena Mortimer, Michele A. O'Connell and Sonia R. Grover
Identifying the Resource Needs of Young People with Differences of Sex Development
Reprinted from: *J. Clin. Med.* **2022**, *11*, 4372, doi:10.3390/jcm11154372 45

Bryan S. Sack, K. Elizabeth Speck, Anastasia L. Hryhorczuk, David E. Sandberg, Kate H. Kraft, Matthew W. Ralls, et al.
An Interdisciplinary Approach to Müllerian Outflow Tract Obstruction Associated with Cloacal Malformation and Cloacal Exstrophy
Reprinted from: *J. Clin. Med.* **2022**, *11*, 4408, doi:10.3390/jcm11154408 55

Lea Tschaidse, Marcus Quinkler, Hedi Claahsen-van der Grinten, Anna Nordenström, Aude De Brac de la Perriere, Matthias K. Auer and Nicole Reisch
Body Image and Quality of Life in Women with Congenital Adrenal Hyperplasia
Reprinted from: *J. Clin. Med.* **2022**, *11*, 4506, doi:10.3390/jcm11154506 65

Susanne Krege, Henrik Falhammar, Hildegard Lax, Robert Roehle, Hedi Claahsen-van der Grinten, Barbara Kortmann, et al.
Long-Term Results of Surgical Treatment and Patient-Reported Outcomes in Congenital Adrenal Hyperplasia—A Multicenter European Registry Study
Reprinted from: *J. Clin. Med.* **2022**, *11*, 4629, doi:10.3390/jcm11154629 79

Verónica Calonga-Solís, Helena Fabbri-Scallet, Fabian Ott, Mostafa Al-Sharkawi, Axel Künstner, Lutz Wünsch, et al.
MYRF: A New Regulator of Cardiac and Early Gonadal Development—Insights from Single Cell RNA Sequencing Analysis
Reprinted from: *J. Clin. Med.* **2022**, *11*, 4858, doi:10.3390/jcm11164858 91

Alice Hoeller, Sahra Steinmacher, Katharina Schlammerl, Markus Hoopmann,
Christl Reisenauer, Valerie Hattermann, et al.
Reassessment of Surgical Procedures for Complex Obstructive Genital Malformations: A Case Series on Different Surgical Approaches
Reprinted from: *J. Clin. Med.* **2022**, *11*, 5026, doi:10.3390/jcm11175026 . . . . **103**

Rebecca Buchert, Elisabeth Schenk, Thomas Hentrich, Nico Weber, Katharina Rall,
Marc Sturm, et al.
Genome Sequencing and Transcriptome Profiling in Twins Discordant for
Mayer-Rokitansky-Küster-Hauser Syndrome
Reprinted from: *J. Clin. Med.* **2022**, *11*, 5598, doi:10.3390/jcm11195598 . . . . **121**

Sahra Steinmacher, Hans Bösmüller, Massimo Granai, André Koch, Sara Yvonne Brucker
and Kristin Katharina Rall
Endometriosis in Patients with Mayer-Rokitansky-Küster- Hauser-Syndrome—Histological Evaluation of Uterus Remnants and Peritoneal Lesions and Comparison to Samples from Endometriosis Patients without Mullerian Anomaly
Reprinted from: *J. Clin. Med.* **2022**, *11*, 6458, doi:10.3390/jcm11216458 . . . . **137**

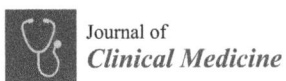

Article

Laparoscopic Vaginoplasty Procedure Using a Modified Peritoneal Pull-Down Technique with Uterine Strand Incision in Patients with Mayer–Rokitansky–Küster–Hauser Syndrome: Kisu Modification

Iori Kisu [1,2,*], Miho Iida [2], Kanako Nakamura [1], Kouji Banno [2], Tetsuro Shiraishi [1], Asahi Tokuoka [1], Keigo Yamaguchi [1], Kunio Tanaka [1], Moito Iijima [1], Hiroshi Senba [1], Kiyoko Matsuda [1] and Nobumaru Hirao [1]

[1] Department of Obstetrics and Gynecology, Federation of National Public Service Personnel Mutual Aid Associations, Tachikawa Hospital, Tokyo 1908531, Japan; konakaramukana0101@hotmail.com (K.N.); shiraishi15@hotmail.co.jp (T.S.); a.tokuoka97@gmail.com (A.T.); tpchkeigo@gmail.com (K.Y.); kunio.tanaka1017@gmail.com (K.T.); moito.not.for.sale@gmail.com (M.I.); semnamik@gmail.com (H.S.); umekiyo@hotmail.co.jp (K.M.); nobumaruhirao@gmail.com (N.H.)
[2] Department of Obstetrics and Gynecology, Keio University School of Medicine, Tokyo 1608582, Japan; mihoiida1029@gmail.com (M.I.); kbanno@keio.jp (K.B.)
* Correspondence: iori71march@hotmail.co.jp or iori71march@a7.keio.jp; Tel.: +81-42-523-3131

Abstract: Various vaginoplasty procedures have been developed for patients with Mayer–Rokitansky–Küster–Hauser (MRKH) syndrome. Here, we describe a novel laparoscopic vaginoplasty procedure, known as the Kisu modification, using a pull-down technique of the peritoneal flaps with additional structural support to the neovaginal apex using the incised uterine strand in patients with MRKH syndrome. Ten patients with MRKH syndrome (mean age at surgery: 23.9 ± 6.5 years, mean postoperative follow-up period: 17.3 ± 3.7 months) underwent construction of a neovagina via laparoscopic vaginoplasty. All surgeries were performed successfully without complications. The mean neovaginal length at discharge was 10.3 ± 0.5 cm. Anatomical success was achieved in all patients, as two fingers were easily introduced, the neovagina was epithelialized, and the mean neovaginal length was 10.1 ± 1.0 cm 1 year postoperatively. No obliteration, granulation tissue formation at the neovaginal apex, or neovaginal prolapse was recorded. Five of the 10 patients attempted sexual intercourse and all five patients were satisfied with the sexual activity, indicating functional success. Although the number of cases in this case series is few, our favorable experience suggests that the Kisu modification of laparoscopic vaginoplasty procedure is an effective, feasible, and safe approach for neovaginal creation in patients with MRKH syndrome.

Keywords: Davydov procedure; Mayer–Rokitansky–Küster–Hauser syndrome; neovagina; uterine factor infertility; uterus transplantation; vaginoplasty; vaginal agenesis

1. Introduction

Mayer–Rokitansky–Küster–Hauser (MRKH) syndrome is a congenital malformation characterized by the defective development of the Müllerian ducts resulting in the absence of a functional vagina and uterus in the presence of normally functioning ovaries. As a result, conception and vaginal sexual activity are compromised. In patients with MRKH syndrome, the creation of a neovagina allows for satisfactory sexual intercourse, and uterus transplantation (UTx) can allow patients with MRKH syndrome to give birth [1].

Several surgical and nonsurgical techniques for creating an adequately sized and functional neovagina to allow for sexual intercourse have been developed for patients with MRKH syndrome [2,3]. However, the surgical method with the best anatomical and functional outcomes is controversial due to a lack of comparative studies [2]. In addition, various materials have been used to cover the newly created space. The laparoscopic Davydov procedure is one of the most commonly used techniques, in which the vesio-rectal

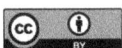

space is coated with peritoneum [4]. However, inadequate pull-down of the peritoneum, obliteration of the neovaginal vault or shortening of the neovagina, granulation tissue formation, and prolapse of the neovagina or bowel are potential limitations of this procedure [2,5,6]. Therefore, various modified laparoscopic Davydov procedures have been developed [6–9].

In this report, we describe a novel laparoscopic vaginoplasty procedure, known as the Kisu modification, using a pull-down technique of the peritoneal flaps with additional structural support to the neovaginal apex using the incised uterine strand (defined as the fibrous band that exists between and connects the bilateral uterine remnants) in patients with MRKH syndrome and report the anatomical and functional outcomes of our case series.

2. Materials and Methods

2.1. Patients

Ten patients with MRKH syndrome underwent neovaginal construction via laparoscopic vaginoplasty at our tertiary hospital. The study was approved by the Institutional Review Board of Federation of National Public Service Personnel Mutual Aid Associations, Tachikawa Hospital, and informed consent was obtained from all patients and/or their parents. All patients with primary amenorrhea underwent pelvic and abdominal ultrasonography, pelvic magnetic resonance imaging, hormonal profiling, and karyotyping to confirm the diagnosis of MRKH syndrome. The patients were counseled regarding the available management options, including surgical and nonsurgical techniques, and patients who chose to undergo a surgical procedure were enrolled in this study. Descriptive results are reported as means and standard deviations (mean ± SD).

2.2. Surgical Procedure

The laparoscopic vaginoplasty procedure used in this case series involved vaginal and laparoscopic approaches (Figures 1–3 and Video S1).

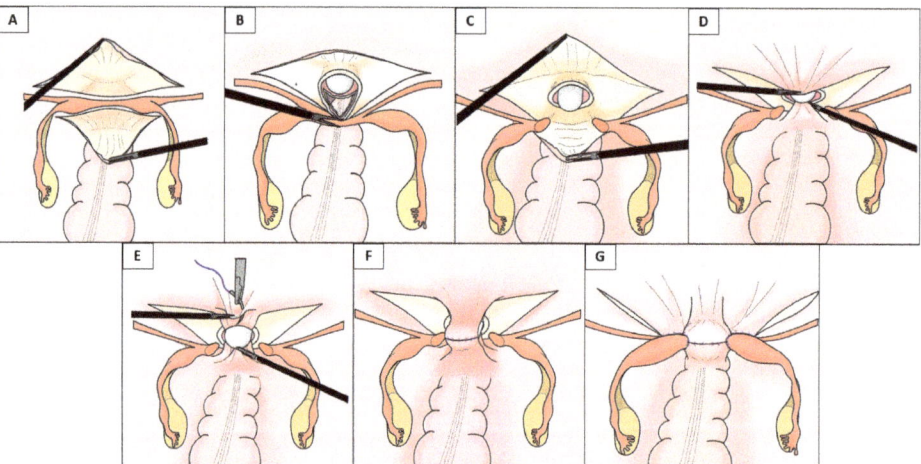

Figure 1. The Kisu modification. This schema shows the laparoscopic creation of a neovagina using a modified peritoneal pull-down technique with uterine strand incision. (**A**) The anterior and posterior peritoneal flaps (the peritoneum in the supravesical pouch and pouch of Douglas) are dissected extensively. (**B**) A transverse incision below the uterine strand serves as the opening of the neovaginal apex. (**C**) The uterine strand is divided via a longitudinal incision. (**D**) The anterior and posterior peritoneal flaps are pulled down through the neovaginal canal and sutured to the neovaginal introitus. (**E**) The neovaginal apex is created by suturing between the supravesical and suprarectal peritoneum at the target neovaginal length. (**F**) The neovaginal apex is shown before suturing the incised uterine strand to the lateral sides of the neovaginal apex. (**G**) The uterine strands provide additional structural support for the neovaginal vault.

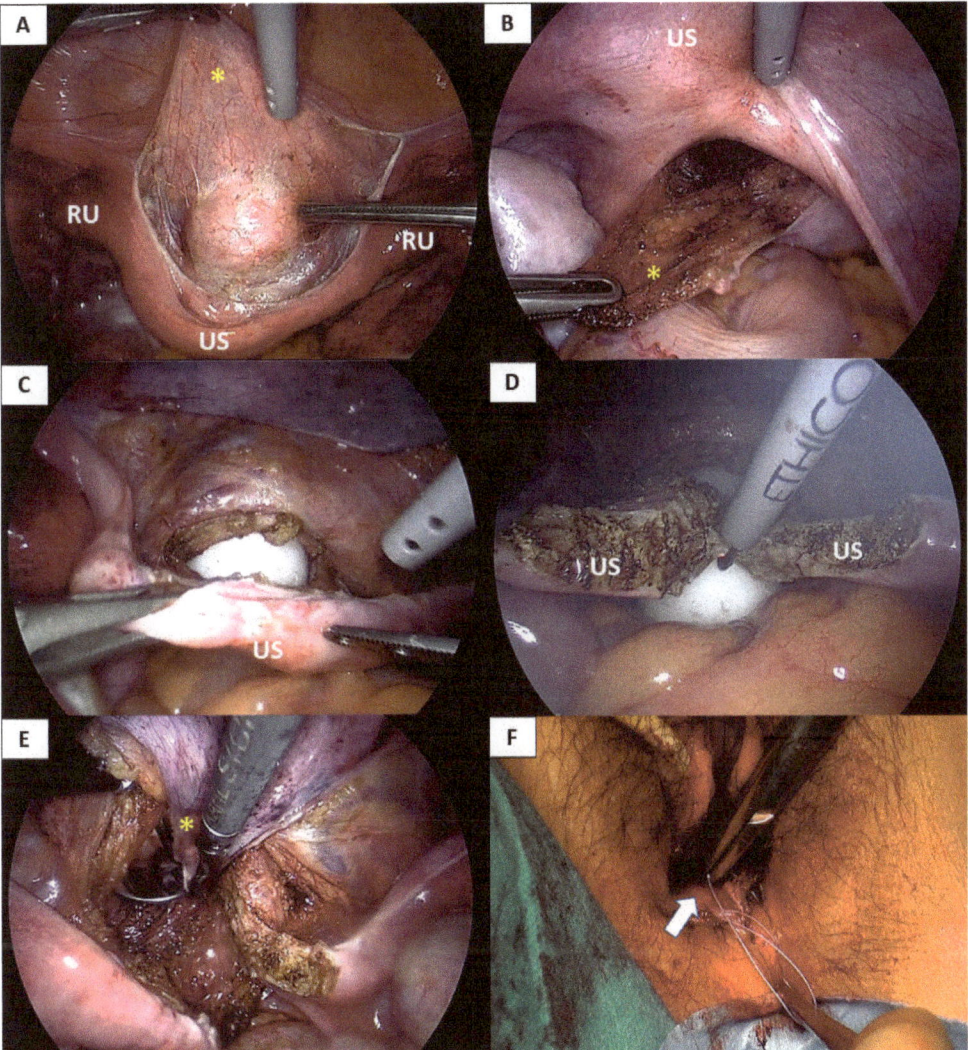

Figure 2. Laparoscopic pull-down technique of the peritoneal flaps with uterine strand incision. (**A**) The supravesical peritoneum (anterior peritoneal flap) (*) along the uterine strand and the bilateral rudimentary uteri is dissected from the bladder. (**B**) The peritoneum of the pouch of Douglas below the uterine strand is incised transversely and mobilized to create the posterior peritoneal flap (*). (**C**) A dilator is inserted through the dissected vaginal space and the apex of the vault is opened with a transverse incision below the strand. (**D**) A longitudinal incision is made in the middle of the uterine strand, dividing the uterine strand bilaterally. (**E**) The edges of the anterior (*) and posterior peritoneal flaps are pulled through the newly created canal under laparoscopic assistance. (**F**) The anterior and posterior flaps are sutured to the anterior and posterior mucosa of the neovaginal introitus. US; Uterine strand, RU; Rudimentary uterus.

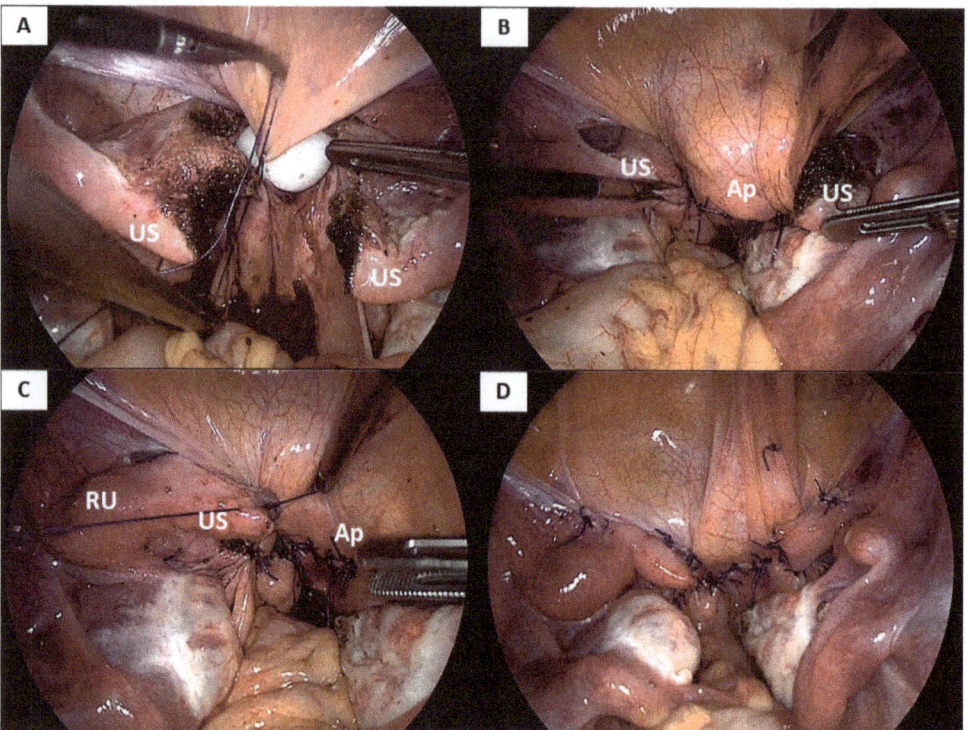

Figure 3. Creation of the neovaginal apex and additional structural support using the incised uterine strand. (**A**) The supravesical and suprarectal peritoneum are sutured at the target neovaginal length while inserting the mold. (**B**) The neovaginal apex is shown with the incised uterine strand before it is used to create additional structural support. (**C**) The incised uterine strand is sutured to the lateral side of the neovaginal apex to cover the side wall of the neovaginal apex and fix the neovaginal canal within the pelvis. (**D**) A final laparoscopic view of the neovaginal apex with the additional structural support created using the incised uterine strand in the Kisu modification technique. US; Uterine strand, RU; Rudimentary uterus, Ap: Apex of the neovagina.

After observing the pelvic and abdominal cavities via laparoscopy, an 8 cm needle was gradually inserted from the vaginal mucosa into the space between the bladder and rectum for injection of normal saline with adrenaline (1:200,000 dilution) to expand the rectovesical space. Then, a 1.5 cm incision was made transversely in the vaginal mucosa followed by gentle blunt dissection into the potential vaginal space between the bladder and rectum to the peritoneum under laparoscopic guidance to maintain the correct direction and avoid injury to the bladder and rectum. The peritoneum of the vesicouterine pouch and pouch of Douglas were mobilized as far as possible for ease of subsequent laparoscopic dissection to create the anterior and posterior flaps for the neovagina.

Following the vaginal approach, a laparoscopic approach was used to dissect the supravesical peritoneum extensively along the uterine strand and the bilateral rudimentary uteri. The peritoneum was dissected from the bladder, allowing the anterior peritoneal flap to be pulled down to the vaginal introitus (Figures 1A and 2A). Next, the uterine strand was lifted, and the peritoneum below the strand (in the pouch of Douglas) was incised transversely, dissected, and mobilized to create the posterior peritoneal flap (Figures 1A and 2B). A 3 cm-wide mold was inserted through the dissected vaginal space and pushed into the vault, the bladder was dissected from the vault, and the apex of the vault was laparoscopically opened via a transverse incision below the uterine strand (Figures 1B and 2C). A longitudinal incision was also made in the middle of the uterine strand, dividing it bilaterally (Figures 1C and 2D). The edges of the separated anterior and posterior flaps were pulled down through the neovaginal canal under laparoscopic assistance and vaginally stitched to the anterior and posterior mucosa of the neovaginal introitus, respectively, using 3-0 absorbable interrupted sutures (Figures 1D and 2E,F). The neovaginal apex was created by suturing the supravesical and suprarectal peritoneum using 1-0 absorbable interrupted sutures at the target neovaginal length (approximately 10 cm) while inserting the mold. The bilateral incised uterine strands were then sutured to the lateral aspects of the neovaginal apex using 1-0 absorbable interrupted or continuous sutures to cover the side wall of the neovaginal apex and fix the neovaginal canal in the pelvis to prevent prolapse of the neovagina (Figures 1F,G and 3C,D). Finally, a methacrylic resin mold was inserted into the neovagina to prevent vaginal stenosis.

3. Results

The patient characteristics and postoperative outcomes shown in Table 1. These patients showed no associated anomalies, including those of the urinary, skeletal and recto-anal systems. One patient had a history of vaginal construction surgery at a different hospital. The mean patient age at surgery was 23.9 ± 6.5 years, and the mean postoperative follow-up period was 17.3 ± 3.7 months. The preoperative vaginal length ranged from absent to 2.5 cm, with the exception of the patient with a history of vaginoplasty who had a vaginal length of 4 cm.

All patients had normally developed external genitalia, bilateral rudimentary uteri, a uterine strand, and normally developed ovaries and Fallopian tubes. A left functional rudimentary uterus was observed in two patients, which was excised. All surgeries were performed successfully without complications. The mean neovaginal length at discharge was 10.3 ± 0.5 cm. Anatomical success was achieved in all patients, as two fingers were easily introduced, the neovagina was epithelialized, and the mean neovaginal length was 10.1 ± 1.0 cm at 1 year postoperatively. No obliteration or granulation tissue formation of the neovaginal apex or neovaginal prolapse was recorded. (Figure 4).

Five patients had a sexual partner and attempted sexual intercourse. Although objective evaluation of a satisfactory sexual life was not performed in this study, these patients were satisfied with their sexual life, indicating functional success. Patients who were not sexually active continued intermittent dilator exercises that maintained an adequate length and neovaginal width (Video S1).

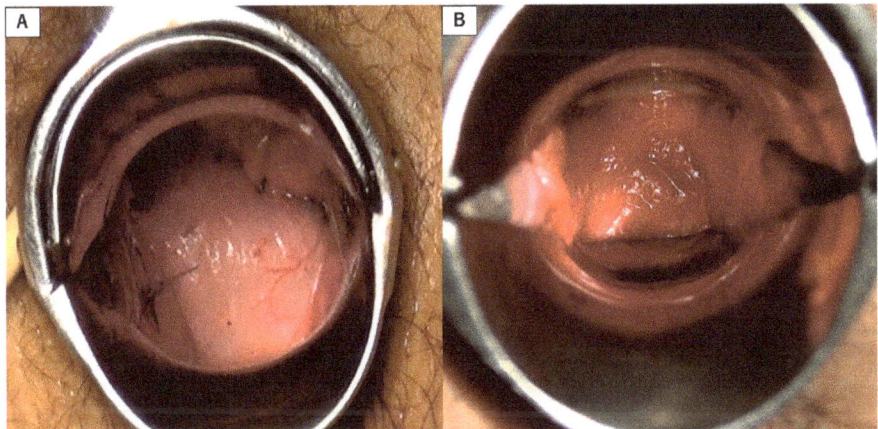

Figure 4. Speculum exam of the apex of the neovagina. (**A**) The neovaginal apex created by suturing the supravesical and suprarectal peritoneum is shown immediately postoperatively. (**B**) The mucosa of the neovagina is epithelialized without granulation tissue formation three months postoperatively.

Table 1. Postoperative outcomes of vaginoplasty in patients.

Case	Age at Surgery	Postoperative Follow-Up Length (Months)	Vaginal Length at Initial Examination (cm)	Neovaginal Length (cm)				Intraoperative Complications	Sexual Activity
				at Discharge	Three Months Postoperatively	6 Months Postoperatively	12 Months Postoperatively		
1	26	24	1	9	8	8	8	No	Satisfactory
2	21	23	Absent	10.5	10.5	10.5	9.5	No	Satisfactory
3	19	15	Absent	10.5	10.5	10	9	No	Satisfactory
4	23	16	Absent	10.5	10.5	10.5	10.5	No	Not attempted
5	34	14	4 *	10.5	11	11.0	10.5	No	Not attempted
6	18	15	Absent	10.5	10	9	9.5	No	Satisfactory
7	16	19	2.5	10.5	11	11	11	No	Not attempted
8	19	19	2	10.5	11	11	11	No	Not attempted
9	36	16	Absent	10.5	10.5	11	11	No	Not attempted
10	27	12	2	10.5	11	11	11	No	Satisfactory
Mean (±SD)	23.9 ± 6.5	17.3 ± 3.7	1.2 ± 1.3	10.3 ± 0.5	10.4 ± 0.9	10.3 ± 1.0	10.1 ± 1.0		

* History of vaginal surgery at an outside hospital.

4. Discussion

This report presents a novel laparoscopic vaginoplasty procedure using a pull-down technique of the peritoneal flaps with extra structural support to the neovaginal apex using the incised uterine strands in 10 patients with MRKH syndrome.

Several nonsurgical and surgical procedures to create a neovagina for patients with MRKH syndrome have been developed. Primary vaginal self-dilation has been recommended as a first-line therapy as it is noninvasive, does not require hospitalization, has minimal complications, and is cost effective [2,3,5,10]. Although this nonsurgical procedure has a high success rate of 74–95% [2,3,11], it is time-consuming and requires strict patient compliance for daily dilation. In addition, dilation therapy may result in comparatively shorter vaginas than surgical procedures [2,3,12].

The surgical procedure that results in the best functional outcome and sexual satisfaction is controversial [2]. There are various surgical techniques for constructing a neovagina, and the choice is always a compromise between the individual needs of each patient and the surgeon's expertise. The Davydov procedure is a classical and effective technique based on pulling down the peritoneum and suturing it to the vaginal introitus. This procedure is safe and easy to perform without the risk of peritoneal flap necrosis or rejection reactions, which are complications of other transferred grafts. Furthermore, epithelialization of the peritoneum begins immediately as the peritoneum has high regenerative powers and can undergo squamous metaplasia when exposed to the external environment, allowing for prompt sexual activity after surgery [6]. However, the Davydov procedure is limited by several potential complications [2,5,6]. Therefore, different methods for the mobilization and the pull-down technique of the pelvic peritoneum have been reported [6–9].

We previously reported a novel laparoscopic vaginoplasty procedure using a pull-down technique of the peritoneal flaps and the peritoneum of the supravesical pouch and pouch of Douglas with a transverse incision below the uterine strand and fixation of the incised uterine strand at the top of the neovagina [8]. This procedure allows the peritoneum to be pulled down to the vaginal introitus more easily and allows for the creation of a longer neovagina. This procedure also prevents stricture of the vaginal apex and prolapse of the neovagina, resulting in successful anatomical and functional outcomes. However, granulation tissue often forms at the neovaginal apex after surgery due to the existence of the strand at the top of the neovagina, and the neovaginal length depends on the position of the uterine strand even if the uterine strand can be placed at a higher level due to mobilization created by the transverse transection of the uterine strand. Therefore, improvements were necessary to achieve an optimal peritoneal vaginoplasty.

The Kisu modification described in this study improves our previously reported laparoscopic vaginoplasty procedure [8]. It consists of mobilization of the extensive anterior and posterior peritoneum in the supravesical pouch and pouch of Douglas, transverse and longitudinal incisions of the uterine strand, creation of the neovaginal apex at the target neovaginal length via suturing between the supravesical and suprarectal peritoneum, and bilateral fixation of the incised uterine strand with the neovaginal apex for additional structural support. This modification allows for the peritoneum to be pulled down to the vaginal introitus adequately and the creation of a neovagina with any length and width without granulation at the apex and prevents vaginal prolapse and perforation due to coitus by reinforcing the apex bilaterally with the incised uterine strand.

The idea of extra structural support using incised uterine strands for the neovaginal vault in Kisu modification was inspired by the recipient surgery of UTx. The first UTx procedure was conducted in Saudi Arabia in 2000, but the transplanted uterus was removed after 99 days because of uterine prolapse with signs of necrosis and vascular thrombosis [13]. This made fixation of the transplanted uterus in the pelvis an important concern, and the method entailing the uterine strand being longitudinally cleaved and incised strands being laterally attached to the transplanted uterus for uterine fixation in the pelvis was developed for the current recipient surgery of UTx in MRKH syndrome [14]. We applied this technique for extra structural support to vaginoplasty to prevent neovaginal prolapse and reinforce the neovaginal apex. Another report also divided the rudimentary uteri to provide further support to the vaginal apex based on the same theory [7].

One potential limitation of the Kisu modification is that adhesions may form between the bladder and rectum as a result of suturing between the supravesical and suprarectal peritoneum. Adhesions may impair the feasibility of future UTx surgery due to altered pelvic anatomical structures. Vaginal dilation is an optimal option when subsequent UTx surgeries are planned [15]. Therefore, injuries to the bladder and rectum should be carefully monitored and avoided when patients plan to undergo UTx. UTx for women with uterine factor infertility is increasing; therefore, the demand for vaginoplasty for patients with MRKH syndrome is expected to increase in the future as the creation of an adequate neovagina is a prerequisite for UTx. As vaginal stenosis after UTx has been reported [16,17], surgical and non-surgical vaginoplasty procedures that can provide sufficient vaginal length and width are important for the reproductive plans of patients with MRKH syndrome.

5. Conclusions

The reported outcomes of these 10 patients suggest that the Kisu modification of the laparoscopic vaginoplasty procedure is an anatomically and functionally effective surgical treatment for patients with MRKH syndrome. While this case series reports relatively few cases, the Kisu modification is a feasible peritoneal vaginoplasty technique that may achieve more optimal outcomes than current techniques for vaginoplasty.

Supplementary Materials: The following is available online at https://www.mdpi.com/article/10.3390/jcm10235510/s1, Video S1: Laparoscopic vaginoplasty procedure using a modified peritoneal pull-down technique with uterine strand incision (Kisu modification).

Author Contributions: Conceptualization, I.K.; methodology, I.K., M.I. (Miho Iida), K.N. and K.B.; investigation, I.K., K.N., T.S., A.T., K.Y., K.T., K.M., M.I. (Moito Iijima) and H.S.; writing—original draft preparation, I.K.; writing—review and editing, M.I. (Miho Iida), K.N., T.S., A.T., K.Y., K.T., K.M., M.I. (Moito Iijima) and N.H.; collecting data, I.K.; supervision, K.B. and N.H. All authors have read and agreed to the published version of the manuscript.

Funding: This research received no external funding.

Institutional Review Board Statement: The study was conducted according to the guidelines of the Declaration of Helsinki and approved by the Institutional Review Board of the Federation of National Public Service Personnel Mutual Aid Associations Tachikawa Hospital (Protocol identification number: 202003).

Informed Consent Statement: Written informed consent was obtained from all subjects involved in the study.

Data Availability Statement: Data are available in a publicly accessible repository.

Conflicts of Interest: The authors declare no conflict of interest.

References

1. Brännström, M.; Johannesson, L.; Bokström, H.; Kvarnström, N.; Mölne, J.; Dahm-Kähler, P.; Enskog, A.; Milenkovic, M.; Ekberg, J.; Diaz-Garcia, C.; et al. Livebirth after uterus transplantation. *Lancet* **2015**, *385*, 607–616. [CrossRef]
2. Callens, N.; De Cuypere, G.; De Sutter, P.; Monstrey, S.; Weyers, S.; Hoebeke, P.; Cools, M. An update on surgical and non-surgical treatments for vaginal hypoplasia. *Hum. Reprod. Update* **2014**, *20*, 775–801. [CrossRef]
3. Cheikhelard, A.; Bidet, M.; Baptiste, A.; Viaud, M.; Fagot, C.; Khen-Dunlop, N.; Louis-Sylvestre, C.; Sarnacki, S.; Touraine, P.; Elie, C.; et al. Surgery is not superior to dilation for the management of vaginal agenesis in Mayer-Rokitansky-Küster-Hauser syndrome: A multicenter comparative observational study in 131 patients. *Am. J. Obstet. Gynecol.* **2018**, *219*, 281.e1–281.e9. [CrossRef]
4. Soong, Y.K.; Chang, F.H.; Lai, Y.M.; Lee, C.L.; Chou, H.H. Results of modified laparoscopically assisted neovaginoplasty in 18 patients with congenital absence of vagina. *Hum. Reprod.* **1996**, *11*, 200–203. [CrossRef] [PubMed]
5. Willemsen, W.N.; Kluivers, K.B. Long-term results of vaginal construction with the use of Frank dilation and a peritoneal graft (Davydov procedure) in patients with Mayer-Rokitansky-Küster syndrome. *Fertil Steril.* **2015**, *103*, 220–227.e1. [CrossRef] [PubMed]

6. Zhao, X.; Wang, R.; Wang, Y.; Li, L.; Zhang, H.; Kang, S. Comparison of two laparoscopic peritoneal vaginoplasty techniques in patients with Mayer-Rokitansky-Küster-Hauser syndrome. *Int. Urogynecol. J.* **2015**, *26*, 1201–1207. [CrossRef] [PubMed]
7. Uncu, G.; Özerkan, K.; Ata, B.; Kasapoğlu, I.; Atalay, M.A.; Orhan, A.; Aslan, K. Anatomic and Functional Outcomes of Paramesonephric Remnant-Supported Laparoscopic Double-Layer Peritoneal Pull-Down Vaginoplasty Technique in Patients with Mayer-Rokitansky-Küster-Hauser Syndrome: Uncu Modification. *J. Minim. Invasive Gynecol.* **2018**, *25*, 498–506. [CrossRef] [PubMed]
8. Kisu, I.; Ito, M.; Nakamura, K.; Shiraishi, T.; Iijima, T.; Senba, H.; Matsuda, K.; Hirao, N. New Laparoscopic Vaginoplasty Procedure With a Modified Peritoneal Pull-Down Technique in Four Patients with Mayer-Rokitansky-Küster-Hauser Syndrome. *J. Pediatr. Adolesc. Gynecol.* **2021**, *34*, 569–572. [CrossRef] [PubMed]
9. Fedele, L.; Frontino, G.; Restelli, E.; Ciappina, N.; Motta, F.; Bianchi, S. Creation of a neovagina by Davydov's laparoscopic modified technique in patients with Rokitansky syndrome. *Am. J. Obstet. Gynecol.* **2010**, *202*, 33.e1–33.e6. [CrossRef] [PubMed]
10. Committee on Adolescent Health Care. ACOG Committee Opinion No. 728: Mullerian Agenesis: Diagnosis, Management, And Treatment. *Obstet. Gynecol.* **2018**, *131*, e35–e42. [CrossRef] [PubMed]
11. Edmonds, D.K.; Rose, G.L.; Lipton, M.G.; Quek, J. Mayer-Rokitansky-Kuster-Hauser syndrome: A review of 245 consecutive cases managed by a multidisciplinary approach with vaginal dilators. *Fertil. Steril.* **2012**, *97*, 686–690. [CrossRef] [PubMed]
12. McQuillan, S.K.; Grover, S.R. Dilation and surgical management in vaginal agenesis: A systematic review. *Int. Urogynecol. J.* **2014**, *25*, 299–311. [CrossRef] [PubMed]
13. Fageeh, W.; Raffa, H.; Jabbad, H.; Marzouki, A. Transplantation of the human uterus. *Int. J. Gynaecol. Obstet.* **2002**, *76*, 245–251. [CrossRef]
14. Brännström, M.; Johannesson, L.; Dahm-Kähler, P.; Enskog, A.; Mölne, J.; Kvarnström, N.; Diaz-Garcia, C.; Hanafy, A.; Lundmark, C.; Marcickiewicz, J.; et al. First clinical uterus transplantation trial: A six-month report. *Fertil Steril.* **2014**, *101*, 1228–1236. [CrossRef] [PubMed]
15. Kölle, A.; Taran, F.A.; Rall, K.; Schöller, D.; Wallwiener, D.; Brucker, S.Y. Neovagina creation methods and their potential impact on subsequent uterus transplantation: A review. *BJOG* **2019**, *126*, 1328–1335. [CrossRef] [PubMed]
16. Chmel, R.; Novackova, M.; Janousek, L.; Matecha, J.; Pastor, Z.; Maluskova, J.; Cekal, M.; Kristek, J.; Olausson, M.; Fronek, J. Revaluation and lessons learned from the first 9 cases of a Czech uterus transplantation trial: Four deceased donor and 5 living donor uterus transplantations. *Am. J. Transplant.* **2019**, *19*, 855–864. [CrossRef] [PubMed]
17. Brännström, M.; Dahm-Kähler, P.; Ekberg, J.; Akouri, R.; Growth, K.; Enskog, A.; Broecker, V.; Mölne, J.; Ayoubi, J.-M.; Kvarnström, N. Outcome of Recipient Surgery and 6-Month Follow-Up of the Swedish Live Donor Robotic Uterus Transplantation Trial. *J. Clin. Med.* **2020**, *9*, 2338. [CrossRef] [PubMed]

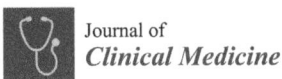

Article

Diagnosis of DSD in Children—Development of New Tools for a Structured Diagnostic and Information Management Program within the Empower-DSD Study

Katja Wechsung [1,*], Louise Marshall [2], Martina Jürgensen [2], Uta Neumann [1,3] and on behalf of the Empower-DSD Study Group [†]

1. Department for Pediatric Endocrinology and Diabetology, Center for Chronic Sick Children, Charité-Universitätsmedizin Berlin, Augustenburger Platz 1, 13353 Berlin, Germany; uta.neumann@charite.de
2. Division of Pediatric Endocrinology and Diabetes, Department of Pediatrics and Adolescent Medicine, University of Lübeck, Ratzeburger Allee 160, 23538 Luebeck, Germany; louise.marshall@uksh.de (L.M.); martina.juergensen@uni-luebeck.de (M.J.)
3. Institute for Experimental Pediatric Endocrinology, Charité-Universitätsmedizin Berlin, Augustenburger Platz 1, 13353 Berlin, Germany
* Correspondence: katja.wechsung@charite.de
† Members of the study group are listed in Appendix A.

Abstract: Background: Current recommendations define a structured diagnostic process, transparent information, and psychosocial support by a specialized, multi-professional team as central in the care for children and adolescents with genital variations and a suspected difference of sex development (DSD). The active involvement of the child and their parents in shared decision-making should result in an individualized care plan. So far, this process has not been standardized. Methods: Within the Empower-DSD study, a team of professionals and representatives of patient advocacy groups developed a new diagnostic and information management program based on current recommendations and existing patient information. Results: The information management defines and standardizes generic care elements for the first weeks after a suspected DSD diagnosis. Three different tools were developed: a guideline for the specialized multiprofessional team, a personal health record and information kit for the child with DSD and their family, and a booklet for medical staff not specialized in DSD. Conclusions: The new information management offers guidance for patients and professionals during the first weeks after a DSD diagnosis is suspected. The developed tools' evaluation will provide further insight into the diagnostic and information-sharing process as well as into all of the involved stakeholders' needs.

Keywords: DSD; information management; shared decision-making; genital variation; gender assignment; diagnostics; standardized care

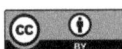

1. Introduction

The acronym DSD (differences of sex development) refers to rare congenital conditions that affect the chromosomal, anatomical, or gonadal sex differentiation [1]. Genital variation is a clinical sign of some DSD diagnoses. It can prompt questions regarding gender assignment and treatment.

Historically, the "optimal gender policy" involved gender assignment to female or male and early surgery to "normalize" genital appearance [2]. Medical professionals made decisions and disclosed little to no information to the affected individuals (paternalistic decision-making). Individuals with DSD have challenged this approach, which profoundly changed the recommendations for care since the beginning of the 21st century [1,3]. Research has highlighted the requirements of children and families for a transparent communication and complete information about the condition [4,5]. Increasingly, genetic mutations are found in the diagnostic process. An exact diagnosis can be made. Evidence for the long-term outcome of medical interventions remains scarce for most DSD conditions. Decisions have to be made on an individual level [6].

Current guidelines therefore propose an informed shared decision-making approach with the active involvement of children and their parents [1,7,8].

Over the course of the shared decision-making process, health care providers and patients collaborate on the way to reach health decisions [9]. This process acknowledges that decisions against the background of uncertain evidence are influenced by the family's emotional, social, and cultural background—likewise also by the health provider's preferences [10]. Important elements of the shared-decision process are the provision of knowledge for the family and the joint discussion of risks and benefits of treatment options [11]. This type of decision-making aims to minimize decisional regret, as well as raise adherence to care and resilience [12].

Thus, education and information transfer are crucial in the care for children with DSD. The DSD-life study has identified information management as a priority of patients to improve care [13]. Information management in the DSD context comprises the information of patients and families by professionals, the information of children by their parents but also the information of the family's social network. A need for "practical resources for patient/caregiver education and decision-making" was also noticed in a study that defined the principles of quality care for pediatric patients with DSD [14]. So far, no standardized information tools exist for children with DSD and their families. An information program that could assist professionals in the condition-specific education of children and their family is lacking.

The first weeks after a suspected DSD diagnosis are critical for children or adolescents and their families. Parents or older children rapidly seek information on the internet, which can be confusing and of poor quality [15,16]. Worries about the child's identity, future perspectives and a wish for a rapid diagnosis can infer a sense of urgency and anxiety [17]. The affected children and parents face a number of challenges to understand the complex aspects of DSD and to find specialized medical as well as psychosocial care that can guide them in decision-making [18].

In Germany, several specialized DSD centers offer a patient/family-centered care by a multidisciplinary team, according to the current recommendations [7,8]. The interdisciplinary team organizes diagnostic procedures, psychosocial support, and transparent information concerning the child and their parents. So far, this information and care process for children and youth with newly diagnosed DSD, which might be associated with genital variation or questions of gender assignment, has not been standardized in Germany.

Within the study Empower-DSD, a structured diagnostic and information management was developed to standardize the care of children during the first weeks after a DSD diagnosis is suspected. On the one hand, the emphasis lies on the provision of existing knowledge on medical, social, legal aspects, and treatment options. On the other hand, the importance of psychosocial care and peer support is taken into account.

The present publication describes the development of the information management and presents the resulting structure, materials, and tools.

The information management addresses children of different age groups (newborn to adolescent child) and their caregivers. The term "family" is used to take into account the various constellations.

2. Methods

2.1. Study Design

Empower-DSD is a prospective longitudinal, mixed methods, non-controlled multicenter study. The study is funded by the German Innovation Fund of health insurance companies.

One objective of the study is to develop and evaluate an information management for children with a newly diagnosed DSD, which is associated with genital ambiguity or questions of gender assignment and their parents. The aim of information management is to foster the diagnosis-specific knowledge and empowerment of patients and their parents, thereby promoting shared decision-making. The information management purports to improve openness and coping with the diagnosis. Thus, the goal is to ensure the affected children's optimal development and enhance patient satisfaction.

The other objective of the Empower DSD study is to develop and evaluate an age-specific group education program for children and adolescents with DSD and their parents [19].

2.2. Study Group

The Empower-DSD study group consists of 14 professionals (psychosocial and medical staff) working in specialized DSD departments of five university hospitals in Germany and representatives of German patient support groups for CAH and XX-/XY-DSD.

The Institute of Social Medicine, Epidemiology and Health Economics (Charité-Universitätsmedizin) is participating in the study for the qualitative evaluation. The Institute of Clinical Epidemiology and Biometry (University of Würzburg) is in charge of the central data management.

2.3. Development of the Information Management

A working group of pediatric endocrinologists and psychosocial professionals from two German DSD centers first developed a list of diagnostic procedures, medical, and psychosocial topics relevant in the first weeks after a DSD diagnosis is suspected.

The two centers' experiences and structures were compared, common elements of care and topics for the information management identified. Initially, two target groups for gathering information (families and professionals) were determined. The group decided on the development of paper-based materials for these two groups. The elements of care concerning the first weeks were arranged in a timeline, the topic list grouped in this order.

The material for professionals was split into two separate items, when it became obvious that the need for information for professionals less experienced in DSD and members of the specialized team differed. The working group therefore decided on a structure in three separate, paper-based materials aiming for the different target groups: families, professionals outside a DSD center, and professionals in a DSD center. Drafts of these documents were prepared and structured according to the initial topic list from October 2019 to March 2020 in the working group. Finally, the material was circulated in the Empower-DSD study group. Further comments and suggestions were discussed and included if relevant. The Empower-DSD study group agreed on a common terminology and the use of an inclusive language, which was applied to all materials.

A consensus meeting with representatives of all study centers (at least one team member with medical and one member with psychosocial background) and patient advocacy groups was held in June 2020 to discuss open questions, organization issues, and, finally, to approve the information management´s structure and content.

2.4. Compilation of Evidence and Existing Materials

A PubMed® search was performed for full-text English language articles using the search terms DSD/diagnostic guideline, DSD/standard, DSD/consensus, DSD/diagnosis, DSD/psychology, DSD/imaging, and DSD/genetics. Guidelines, consensus statements, and reviews published from 2010 to 2020 as well as relevant articles from the reference lists of those were selected.

The information management includes existing patient information. To obtain an overview of existing materials, an open-hand and online search were conducted. First, existing print patient brochures for families with newly diagnosed DSD used in the DSD centers were reviewed. Second, available print material (brochures and information leaflets that are downloadable as pdf) was searched online in January 2020 and again in March 2022 via Google using the search terms "DSD", "Varianten der Geschlechtsentwicklung" ("variants of sexual development"), "intersex", "AGS", and "CAH". The first 100 search results were considered. Materials were integrated if they were written in German, contained medical and/or psychosocial information relevant for the first weeks after a suspected DSD diagnosis with genital variation or questions of gender assignment and fulfilled the EQIP criteria for quality [20]. Moreover, the working group screened material in English for additional topics not yet incorporated in German brochures.

2.5. Evaluation of the Information Management

The developed information management will be evaluated. Children with suspected XX-/XY-DSD as well as sex chromosomal DSD and their surrogates with first appointments in four participating DSD clinics (Berlin, Lübeck, Bochum, Ulm) will be offered participation in the evaluation. The study aims for the inclusion of 30 children/adolescents and their parents.

For the quantitative evaluation, the diagnosis, the included patients' age, and the information management process's documentation will be analyzed with descriptive statistics. A qualitative evaluation with semi-structured interviews of the patients, their families, professionals, and peers will assess the expectations as well as hopes for the information management and how the participation was experienced. The evaluation will be performed after all included patients have completed the information management program. There is no interim analysis planned.

3. Results

The Empower-DSD information management organizes the diagnostic and information process for primary and specialized care after a suspected DSD diagnosis.

The materials' medical and psychosocial information is based on national and international consensus statements, published expert opinions, and results of DSD research. In a literature search via PubMed®, 26 articles were retrieved. Twelve guidelines and general care recommendations were identified [7,8,13,20–28]. Moreover, articles with a special focus on the somatic, biochemical, and genetic assessment, as well as on imaging and psychosocial care in children with a suspected DSD diagnosis, were selected [29–42].

In the search for existing patient information, seven materials directed to parents and children were found. Four materials were selected to be passed on to the families during the information management (Table S1). All included brochures covered topics related to a diagnosis in the newborn period. No information directed toward older children and their parents was found. There was only one booklet addressing health care professionals, i.e., obstetricians. It contained specific guidance for the communication with parents of newborn children. No material including communication skills with older children for primary care providers was identified. During the study, the web page https://dsdcare.de (accessed on 16 May 2022) was launched providing insightful information about existing materials for families in Germany.

Within the Empower-DSD study, three new paper-based tools were developed, addressing the needs of the different target groups that are involved in the diagnosis and care process:

One tool was created for staff not specialized in DSD. It provides general information about the first contact and the time until referral to a specialized DSD center. In addition, it includes a list of existing patient brochures. Two tools assist the care in the specialized DSD center: "My record", a personal health record and information kit for the child/youth with DSD and their family; a guideline for the specialized multidisciplinary team containing templates with a checklist that aid the standardization as well as documentation of the information transfer to the family. Figure 1 illustrates the defined elements of care and information management tools. The following overview will outline the care process defined by the developed materials. It will introduce the new tools and their use in more detail.

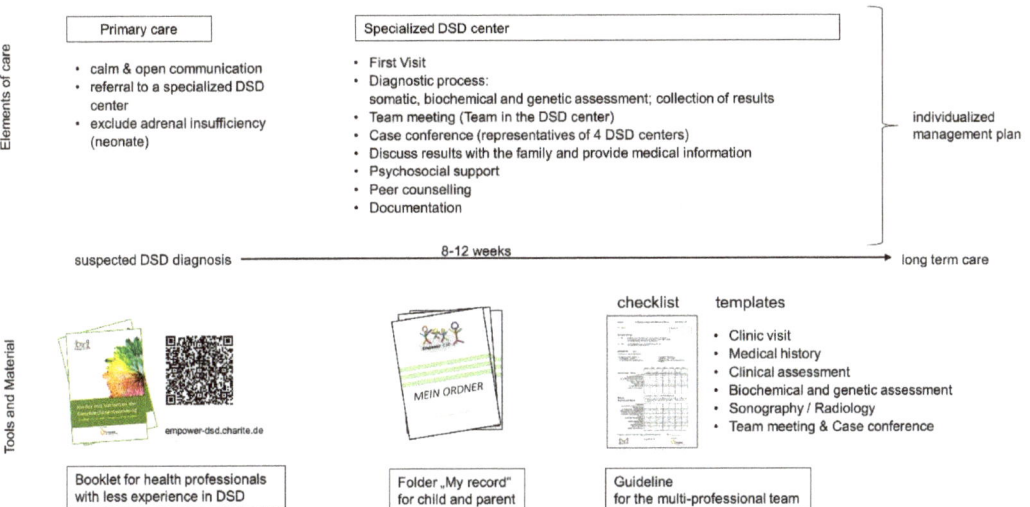

Figure 1. Elements of care and developed tools of the information management.

3.1. A booklet for the First Contact in Primary Care

The suspicion of a DSD diagnosis mostly arises in a primary care setting. Genital variation at birth, absent pubertal development, or the incidental finding of abdominal gonads during surgery are examples where professionals like pediatricians, neonatologists, gynecologists, urologists, pediatric surgeons, midwifes, and nurses could suspect a DSD diagnosis in a child or adolescent. To address health care professionals with less experience in the treatment of DSD, a short 18-page booklet (written in German) was developed. The booklet is meant to provide an overview on important topics for this early period. The document aims to facilitate a calm environment for the family, minimize anxiety, and ensure rapid access to specialized care. In addition, it reassures professionals that the referral to a specialized center is an important step in the care process for children with these rare diagnoses. It advises the avoidance of unnecessary medical procedures. The booklet proposes an open, adequate communication with the families, and gives examples of useful phrases. It refers to existing brochures for parents with newborn children (Table S1).

Table 1 shows a summary of the main topics that are included in the booklet. Information regarding the latter was distributed via the German national societies for pediatrics, gynecology, neonatology, and midwives. It is accessible via the Empower-DSD webpage (https://empower-dsd.charite.de, accessed on 16 May 2022).

Table 1. Content of the booklet for health care professionals outside the specialized DSD center.

- Medical background: What does the acronym DSD stand for?
- Why is the referral to a specialized center important?
- How quickly should a referral happen?—Urgent diagnostic procedures are only important to exclude CAH and other forms of adrenal insufficiency in the newborn.
- Guide for the communication with parents of newborn and older children/adolescents including useful phrases and wording.
- Contact to specialized centers and newborn screening labs in Germany.
- Contact to patient support groups and a list of existing patient information brochures.

3.2. Guideline and Checklist for the Specialized DSD Center

The guideline for the specialized multidisciplinary team defines structural requirements for the information management in the specialized DSD center. The multidisciplinary team should encompass pediatric endocrinology, psychology, pediatric radiology, and surgical subspecialty (pediatric surgery and/or pediatric gynecology and/or pediatric urology). Other disciplines can be involved as needed (e.g., social work, genetics, ethics, pediatric neurology).

Concerning each care element, the guideline specifies actions for the team and topics that should be discussed with the families. A checklist condenses all elements and corresponding topics (Table 2).

Table 2. Checklist for the Empower-DSD information management.

First Visit			Date: _____	
Check with x if completed, otherwise leave blank				
o explain goals of information management;			o introduce team members;	o concept of psychosocial care;
o concept of peer counselling;			o hand out "My record";	o outline diagnostic process
Date	Date	Date		

Diagnostic process
x—completed; o—not completed; xx—previously performed; n—not applicable

			Medical history
			Somatic assessment
			Biochemical and genetic assessment
			Sonography/imaging
			Referral gynecology
			Referral urology
			Referral pediatric surgery

Diagnosis
c—confirmed; u—unclear; s—suspected

Discuss results; medical information
x—topic discussed; o—not discussed; n—not applicable

			Basics: Sex development, gonads, steroid hormones
			Urgency or non-urgency of treatment
			Development of gender identity
			Expected somatic development
			Options for hormone treatment in puberty
			Individual decision-making
			Fertility
			Malignant potential
			Sexuality
			Risks and benefits of surgery
			Management plan

Psychosocial care parents
x—topic discussed; o—not discussed; n—not applicable

			Address questions, fears, and concerns
			Adopt a positive perspective on the child´s future
			Each family has a different way to approach DSD.
			Recommend the documentation of the decision-making process
			View of biological sex and gender as continua
			Diversity of physical appearance
			Sex assignment
			Communication within the social network (education and disclosure)
			Communication with the healthcare system
			Explaining DSD to the child in an age-appropriate way

Table 2. *Cont.*

Psychosocial care child			
x—topic discussed; o—not discussed; n—not applicable			
			Address questions, fears and concerns
			Adopt a positive perspective on the future
			Education about the child´s body and condition
			Diversity of physical appearance
			Communication within the social network (education and disclosure)
			Explain procedures in the specialized center
			Explain care and guidance over time
			Social and legal issues
			Peer counselling
Team meeting/Case conference (Professions of the attending participants and centers present are documented.)			
x—topic discussed; o—not discussed; n—not applicable			
			Results of assessments
			Urgency of treatment
			Evidence for recommendations
			Management plan
Feedback to referring primary care provider			Date: _____

Each clinic's multidisciplinary team complies with the structural requisites specified in the guideline and documents all consultations as well as discussed topics in the checklist with the current date.

The results of all assessments are shared with the family. To understand the health implications of the DSD diagnosis, the family is educated about sexual development and medical aspects. The child is involved in the information exchange in an age-appropriate manner. The team further addresses psychosocial as well as legal and administrative issues. In consultations with a surgical subspecialty, the risks and benefits of surgical procedures are discussed, if applicable. The family is educated about the options of surgical decision-making according to the change in German legislation from 2021. Surgical interventions on genitals must be deferred until the child can give informed consent, unless the surgery is life-saving. If a surgery is aimed to prevent harm to the child´s health or in case of a sinus urogenitalis in girls with CAH, approval for an early surgery must be requested at the family court.

The guideline defines a duration of eight to twelve weeks after the referral to the DSD clinic for the information management. All relevant topics of the checklist should be discussed at least once, preferably as often as the family requires within this period. However, the checklist does not specify the number of appointments or the sequence of care elements. The team should schedule appointments according to the family's needs. Depending on the location of the DSD service in a rural or urban area and the distance to the family's residence, appointments are made more or less frequently in each center.

A case manager, who is the primary contact for the family organizes the appointments and diagnostic procedures. The case manager´s professional background varies between the DSD centers of the Empower-DSD study group (e.g., pediatric endocrinology, psychology or nurse practitioner). The guideline for the specialized team defines the topics, which have to be discussed with the family. A medical expert covers medical topics and a team member with psychosocial background discusses psychosocial topics with the family.

3.3. My Record

In the specialized center, the case manager introduces the team members and explains the information management's goals and process to the family. The team addresses the family's questions, explains results of earlier investigations, if applicable, and outlines the planned examinations as well as diagnostic procedures. In due course, the team explains the challenges of decision-making in DSD, the purpose of psychosocial care, and potential peer counseling opportunities. If desired, a consultation appointment or meeting with a peer is organized. The team members describe the importance of the diagnostic and decision-making process documentation. The folder named "My record" is handed to the family. The sections are explained (Table 3). "My record" is a paper-based resource kit that combines a personal health record with information on key age-related topics in DSD. This tool is directed at the family (i.e., parents of a younger child) or older child/young adult. Therefore, it is written in a non-technical language. It provides guidance during the information management and beyond for life-long care. The folder can be adapted individually. If updates arise, the team and the family can easily rearrange or replace the paper prints within the folder or add further information.

Table 3. Sections and content of "My record".

Sections and Content	Purpose
Introduction: Welcome letter to the family (different version for parents of a newborn and families with an older child).	Personal Health record
Contact/Appointments: Address, names of the multidisciplinary team members, space to note appointments	
Visit in the DSD clinic: What to expect during the visits at the DSD clinic. Template for taking notes during the visit or preparing questions for the next visit (for professionals and/or patients). What is a team meeting or a case conference? Role of photographs in the somatic assessment.	
Results: Short description of common diagnostic procedures in the DSD clinic and encouragement of the family to keep and file all results/discharge notes here.	
Peer Counseling: Introduction and contact to support groups, explanation of peer counseling.	Information
Medical and psychosocial information: Structured by age. Glossary of medical terms. Brochures of patient support groups designed for families with a recent diagnosis.	
Thoughts and feelings: Place for parents to write down thoughts, feelings, or information regarding the diagnosis process or DSD. This might be a diary entry or a letter to the child. For older children or adolescents, place for own thoughts or feelings.	Documentation of the decision-making process

The folder purports to favor medical information collection. Therefore, there are sections in which to file the results of medical assessments. The documentation in "My record" aims to assist the open discussion of all results and the transition of adolescents to adult care in the further course.

One section provides information on the proceedings during visits in the clinic and a template to take notes. This section's covering page contains a short explanation on possible medical assessments and prepares the family for the next visits.

The information given in "My record" is structured chronologically, addressing questions that might arise during the newborn period (e.g., naming/sex assignment), extending to topics in kindergarten and later during the school career, puberty, and adolescence. This information timeline gives parents a short overview on medical and psychosocial issues in DSD that are important in the present or may be more relevant when the child is older (" *How can I support my child regarding psychosexual development, sexuality and relationships, fertility, gender and society, social network, kindergarten, school, bullying, hobbies, personal strengths, and legal aspects?*"). Families are informed that results of investigations can remain pending for a long time. They are also educated regarding the fact that a genetic diagnosis may not always be made. The chapter explains that medical intervention and non-intervention are equally important in the care of children with DSD.

Parents can use the written information to formulate questions for the team and comprehend the concept of a long-term care process. Existing brochures developed by patient support groups and contact details for peer counselling are filed in a separate section.

The last section, "thoughts and feelings", provides a space for parents of newborn or small children to collect memories about family values, information, and personal thoughts that played a role in their decision-making. This documentation can assist the passing of information from parents to children in an age-appropriate manner. Adolescents are encouraged to keep a diary for thoughts regarding their condition.

3.4. Templates for the Diagnostic Process and Team Meetings

To harmonize the diagnostic process in all study centers, the guidelines for the multi-professional team contain six templates, which can further aid the results' documentation and discussion with the family. The templates summarize recent recommendations on medical history taking, physical examination, and biochemical and genetic assessments, as well as imaging. A photo documentation during the somatic assessment is not required and only possible after the family has given informed consent. Where photographs are stored must be explicitly discussed with the family. Ideally, a copy is placed in "My record".

A template for the clinic visit's documentation can help to retain an overview about who was present, which examinations were performed, and what topics were discussed. This template is included in the guideline for the team as well as in "My record" for the family.

A meeting of the multi-professional team in the specialized center is mandatory in order to discuss the assessments´ results for each patient and to develop a management plan. Furthermore, a case conference with a medical and psychosocial representative of each study center takes place every three months during the study. In these meetings, the team exchanges and collects information on assessments and explores the evidence for recommendations. A template that lists important topics for the team discussion was developed. Results of the team meeting and case conference are discussed with the family. Information on the proceeding of team meetings and the case conference are also included in "My record" for the family.

3.5. Exchange of Information between Primary and Specialized Care

The guideline proposes a feedback concerning the diagnostic procedures' results to the referring and further treating primary care physicians. This report also includes recommendations for further care and treatment. In many cases, joint care is provided, in which families present to the DSD center at specific intervals but are primarily seen by a family physician, pediatrician, or pediatric endocrinologist locally. This requires a good transfer of all necessary information.

3.6. Patient Recruitment

The patient recruitment started in summer 2020. Thirty children/adolescents and their parents started the information management according to the developed materials. Ten families are still in the procedure of completing the checklist and several interviews for qualitative evaluation are outstanding.

4. Discussion

The Empower-DSD information management provides a new standardized information and care program for the first weeks after a suspected DSD diagnosis for children with genital variation and their parents. The structured care process is made transparent to all involved stakeholders via two tools in the specialized DSD center: guidelines and checklist for the multi-professional team and a personal health record for the families ("My record"). The link to primary care is endorsed with a third tool: a booklet for professionals outside a specialized DSD center.

The developed materials disclose relevant information to each target group and thereby support the family's navigation through the medical system. To our knowledge, this is the first standardized program that equally addresses families and professionals.

The variability of DSD conditions—even with the same genotype—makes the use of a clinical algorithm difficult. Parents differ in their needs and ethical/social understanding of gender. Each family has different concepts of what is normal and how to deal with sexuality [6]. The requirements of children change with age [43]. To address this complexity in care, an individualized approach is necessary. Nevertheless, generic elements that recur in the care and education of families with a new DSD diagnosis were identified and sorted in a checklist. The medicalization of DSD is a point of criticism [44]. Psychosocial information is often perceived as missing by parents [45]. The checklist therefore equally values medical and psychosocial aspects of the care process.

The target groups' varying demands were a challenge in the materials' development. While specialists tend to wish for detailed information, parents wish for time to get used to the diagnosis and for practical information regarding daily life [46,47]. To address the different viewpoints of clinicians and individuals with DSD as well as their surrogates, patient support groups were actively included in the developmental process.

Several decision aids for families with newly diagnosed DSD have recently been developed. They focus on the decision-making of parents with newborn children and genital or gonadal surgery [48–51]. Three decision aids consist of checklists for the specialized DSD team. They include lists of topics to discuss with the family. One group developed a complex online tool for the families to navigate at home. Interestingly, this tool was only used by 40% of the families past the first log-in [49]. As one reason, the authors suspected technical problems but also different needs for the depth of information in different families. The information management of Empower-DSD aims to promote informed decision-making by providing education on decision-making and DSD. However, it cannot be seen as a decision-making aid, but as a toolkit to promote information exchange and standardized care. In doing so, it acknowledges that final decisions may or may not be made within the first few weeks.

German legislation banned cosmetic genital surgery on children with a DSD diagnosis in March 2021 and thereby changed the available options for families [52]. Surgery is still possible in life-threatening situations or in special cases after the authorization of a family court (e.g., sinus urogenitalis in CAH females). In all other cases, the decision for surgery must be deferred until an age where the child can participate in decision-making processes.

The information management's contents were split into three separate tools. The latter were meant to provide only relevant information to each target group and avoid information overload. The structure of the information management is flexible and can be adapted to different DSD diagnoses, age groups, and clinic settings. All activities of the multidisciplinary team are documented, which is supposed to support the transition from pediatric to adult health care and thereby improve long-term health. A standardized documentation might also facilitate data entry into registries, as is increasingly demanded concerning rare diseases [24].

The developed materials are designed to be used in an interactive matter at the DSD clinic. The team can review information together with the family and tailor it to the patient's and family's needs. Depending on the family's health literacy, information can be limited to basics or further resources can be shared.

The written information in "My record" complements face-to-face contact. Conversations with the team should extend the information and adapt it to the family's cultural and educational background. The guideline to the DSD team is directed at professionals with experience in communication with families and children with DSD conditions. Research shows that the health provider's communication skills affect parents' decision-making processes [53]. These skills vary wildly, even amongst DSD specialists [54]. While the developed tool for professionals outside the DSD center encompasses tips on how to communicate with the family, no advice on this matter was included in the material for the multi-professional team in the DSD center. Details regarding communication for DSD specialists could be added to the information management in the future.

An effort has been made to integrate existing materials from German support groups into the information management. US and English patient support groups have created resources with reassuring information, such as dsdfamilies.org and the Handbook for Parents (Table S1), which were not included because of the language barrier for the families. The previous project dsd-LIFE translated one brochure designed by dsdfamilies.org into German. Further collaboration in this style could improve the information of families with a new DSD diagnosis. On the other hand, cultural background, health systems, and national judicial regulations differ between the countries, which might impede the adaptation of international materials.

The approach to diagnostics and care in DSD is changing continuously. Ongoing research is to be expected [55]. Information quickly becomes outdated. As mentioned above, the German legislation regarding genital surgery changed since the information management´s first draft. Patient support groups reorganized and updated brochures, accordingly. Hence, materials and tools must be updated on a regular basis. This might be a barrier to the implementation of the developed tools in routine care. On the other hand, "My record" and the checklist are flexible. They can easily be adapted to changing guidelines or local requirements.

5. Conclusions

The newly developed information management for children with a recent DSD diagnosis standardizes the diagnostic and information process for patients, their families and professionals in three paper-based materials. It adapts the information to the families' needs and to the health staff with different degrees of specialization. The materials navigate families through the medical system and endorse the documentation of the care process.

The information management's evaluation will provide deeper insight into the needs and wishes of families and professionals during the first weeks of care.

Supplementary Materials: The following supporting information can be downloaded at: https://www.mdpi.com/article/10.3390/jcm11133859/s1, Table S1: existing information resources.

Author Contributions: Conceptualization, K.W., L.M., M.J. and U.N.; methodology, K.W., L.M., M.J. and U.N.; writing—original draft preparation, K.W.; writing—review and editing, U.N. and Empower-DSD Study Group; visualization, K.W.; supervision, U.N.; project administration, U.N. and Empower-DSD Study Group; funding acquisition, U.N. and Empower-DSD Study Group. All authors have read and agreed to the published version of the manuscript.

Funding: This research was funded by the innovation fund of the German Federal Joint Committee (GBA), grant number 01VSF18022.

Institutional Review Board Statement: The study was conducted in accordance with the Declaration of Helsinki and approved by the Ethics Committee of the leading study center Charité-Universitätsmedizin Berlin (EA2/238/19; 4 March 2020). All participating study centers obtained ethical approval from their institutions.

Informed Consent Statement: Informed consent was obtained from all subjects involved in the study.

Data Availability Statement: Not applicable.

Acknowledgments: Our greatest tribute goes to Birgit Köhler, who worked at the Charité in Berlin and was this study's initiator. She authored the proposal's first draft but passed away before this project started. We appreciate the commitment of the patient support groups and their representatives: AGS-Eltern- und Patienteninitiative e.V. with Manuela Brösamle, Intergeschlechtliche Menschen e.V. (IMeV) with Charlotte Wunn, SHG Interfamilien with Gerda Janssen-Schmidchen, 47xxy Klinefelter Syndrom e.V. with Bernhard Köpl and Dirk Müller, Turner-Syndrom-Vereinigung Deutschland e.V. with Katrin Stahl.

Conflicts of Interest: The authors declare no conflict of interest. The funders had no role in the design of the study; in the collection, analyses, or interpretation of data; in the writing of the manuscript, or in the decision to publish the results.

Appendix A

Empower DSD study group: Manuela Brösamle (AGS-Eltern- und Patienteninitiative e.V.), Martina Ernst (Charité-Universitätsmedizin Berlin), Gloria Herrmann (Universitätsklinikum Ulm), Olaf Hiort (University of Lübeck), Loretta Ihme (Charité-Universitätsmedizin Berlin), Gerda Janssen-Schmidchen (SHG Interfamilien), Ute Kalender (Charité-Universitätsmedizin Berlin), Thomas Keil (Charité-Universitätsmedizin Berlin and University of Würzburg), Bernhard Köpl (47xxy klinefelter syndrom e.v.), Klaus-Peter Liesenkötter (Endokrinologikum Berlin), Annette Richter-Unruh (Ruhr-University Bochum), Julia Rohayem (University Hospital Münster), Stephanie Roll (Charité-Universitätsmedizin Berlin), Ralph Schilling (Charité-Universitätsmedizin Berlin), Julia Schneidewind (University of Lübeck), Katrin Stahl (Turner-Syndrom-Vereinigung Deutschland e.V.), Barbara Stöckigt (Charité-Universitätsmedizin Berlin), Martin Wabitsch (Universitätsklinikum Ulm), Isabel Viola Wagner (University of Lübeck), Sabine Wiegmann (Charité-Universitätsmedizin Berlin), Charlotte Wunn (Intergeschlechtliche Menschen e.V.).

References

1. Lee, P.A.; Houk, C.P.; Ahmed, S.F.; Hughes, I.A.; International Consensus Conference on Intersex organized by the Lawson Wilkins Pediatric Endocrine Society; the European Society for Paediatric Endocrinology. Consensus statement on management of intersex disorders. International Consensus Conference on Intersex. *Pediatrics* **2006**, *118*, e488–e500. [CrossRef]
2. Money, J.; Hampson, J.G.; Hampson, J.L. Hermaphroditism: Recommendations concerning assignment of sex, change of sex and psychologic management. *Bull. Johns Hopkins Hosp.* **1955**, *97*, 284–300. [PubMed]
3. Kemp, B.D. Sex, lies and androgen insensitivity syndrome. *Can. Med. Assoc. J.* **1996**, *154*, 1829, author reply 1833. [PubMed]
4. Lundberg, T.; Lindstrom, A.; Roen, K.; Hegarty, P. From Knowing Nothing to Knowing What, How and Now: Parents' Experiences of Caring for their Children With Congenital Adrenal Hyperplasia. *J. Pediatr. Psychol.* **2017**, *42*, 520–529. [CrossRef] [PubMed]
5. Simoes, E.; Sokolov, A.N.; Kronenthaler, A.; Hiltner, H.; Schäeffeler, N.; Rall, K.; Ueding, E.; Rieger, M.A.; Wagner, A.; Poesch, L.S.; et al. Information ranks highest: Expectations of female adolescents with a rare genital malformation towards health care services. *PLoS ONE* **2017**, *12*, e0174031. [CrossRef]
6. Lampalzer, U.; Briken, P.; Schweizer, K. 'That decision really was mine ... '. Insider perspectives on health care controversies about intersex/diverse sex development. *Cult. Health Sex.* **2021**, *23*, 472–483. [CrossRef]
7. Lee, P.A.; Nordenstrom, A.; Houk, C.P.; Ahmed, S.F.; Auchus, R.; Baratz, A.; Baratz Dalke, K.; Liao, L.M.; Lin-Su, K.; Looijenga, L.H., 3rd; et al. Global Disorders of Sex Development Update since 2006: Perceptions, Approach and Care. *Horm. Res. Paediatr.* **2016**, *85*, 158–180. [CrossRef]
8. Krege, S.; Eckoldt, F.; Richter-Unruh, A.; Kohler, B.; Leuschner, I.; Mentzel, H.J.; Moss, A.; Schweizer, K.; Stein, R.; Werner-Rosen, K.; et al. Variations of sex development: The first German interdisciplinary consensus paper. *J. Pediatr. Urol.* **2019**, *15*, 114–123. [CrossRef]
9. Charles, C.; Gafni, A.; Whelan, T. Shared decision-making in the medical encounter: What does it mean? (or it takes at least two to tango). *Soc. Sci. Med.* **1997**, *44*, 681–692. [CrossRef]
10. Politi, M.C.; Street, R.L., Jr. The importance of communication in collaborative decision making: Facilitating shared mind and the management of uncertainty. *J. Eval. Clin. Pract.* **2011**, *17*, 579–584. [CrossRef]
11. Crissman, H.P.; Warner, L.; Gardner, M.; Carr, M.; Schast, A.; Quittner, A.L.; Kogan, B.; Sandberg, D.E. Children with disorders of sex development: A qualitative study of early parental experience. *Int. J. Pediatr. Endocrinol.* **2011**, *2011*, 10. [CrossRef] [PubMed]
12. Lorenzo, A.J.; Pippi Salle, J.L.; Zlateska, B.; Koyle, M.A.; Bagli, D.J.; Braga, L.H. Decisional regret after distal hypospadias repair: Single institution prospective analysis of factors associated with subsequent parental remorse or distress. *J. Urol.* **2014**, *191*, 1558–1563. [CrossRef]
13. Thyen, U.; Ittermann, T.; Flessa, S.; Muehlan, H.; Birnbaum, W.; Rapp, M.; Marshall, L.; Szarras-Capnik, M.; Bouvattier, C.; Kreukels, B.P.C.; et al. Quality of health care in adolescents and adults with disorders/differences of sex development (DSD) in six European countries (dsd-LIFE). *BMC Health Serv. Res.* **2018**, *18*, 527. [CrossRef] [PubMed]
14. Kavanaugh, G.L.; Mohnach, L.; Youngblom, J.; Kellison, J.G.; Sandberg, D.E.; Accord, A. "Good practices" in pediatric clinical care for disorders/differences of sex development. *Endocrine* **2021**, *73*, 723–733. [CrossRef] [PubMed]
15. Ernst, M.M.; Chen, D.; Kennedy, K.; Jewell, T.; Sajwani, A.; Foley, C.; Sandberg, D.E.; Workgroup, D.-T.P.; Accord, A. Disorders of sex development (DSD) web-based information: Quality survey of DSD team websites. *Int. J. Pediatr. Endocrinol.* **2019**, *2019*, 1. [CrossRef]
16. Shoureshi, P.S.; Rajasegaran, A.; Kokorowski, P.; Sparks, S.S.; Seideman, C.A. Social media engagement, perpetuating selected information, and accuracy regarding CA SB-201: Treatment or intervention on the sex characteristics of a minor. *J. Pediatr. Urol.* **2021**, *17*, 372–377. [CrossRef]
17. Pasterski, V.; Mastroyannopoulou, K.; Wright, D.; Zucker, K.J.; Hughes, I.A. Predictors of posttraumatic stress in parents of children diagnosed with a disorder of sex development. *Arch. Sex. Behav.* **2014**, *43*, 369–375. [CrossRef]
18. Bennecke, E.; Werner-Rosen, K.; Thyen, U.; Kleinemeier, E.; Lux, A.; Jurgensen, M.; Gruters, A.; Kohler, B. Subjective need for psychological support (PsySupp) in parents of children and adolescents with disorders of sex development (dsd). *Eur. J. Pediatr.* **2015**, *174*, 1287–1297. [CrossRef]
19. Wiegmann, S.; Ernst, M.; Ihme, L.; Wechsung, K.; Kalender, U.; Stockigt, B.; Richter-Unruh, A.; Vogler, S.; Hiort, O.; Jurgensen, M.; et al. Development and evaluation of a patient education programme for children, adolescents, and young adults with differences of sex development (DSD) and their parents: Study protocol of Empower-DSD. *BMC Endocr. Disord.* **2022**, *22*, 166. [CrossRef]

20. Moult, B.; Franck, L.S.; Brady, H. Ensuring quality information for patients: Development and preliminary validation of a new instrument to improve the quality of written health care information. *Health Expect.* **2004**, *7*, 165–175. [CrossRef]
21. Moran, M.E.; Karkazis, K. Developing a multidisciplinary team for disorders of sex development: Planning, implementation, and operation tools for care providers. *Adv. Urol.* **2012**, *2012*, 604135. [CrossRef] [PubMed]
22. Kyriakou, A.; Dessens, A.; Bryce, J.; Iotova, V.; Juul, A.; Krawczynski, M.; Nordenskjold, A.; Rozas, M.; Sanders, C.; Hiort, O.; et al. Current models of care for disorders of sex development—results from an International survey of specialist centres. *Orphanet J. Rare Dis.* **2016**, *11*, 155. [CrossRef] [PubMed]
23. Ahmed, S.F.; Achermann, J.C.; Arlt, W.; Balen, A.; Conway, G.; Edwards, Z.; Elford, S.; Hughes, I.A.; Izatt, L.; Krone, N.; et al. Society for Endocrinology UK guidance on the initial evaluation of an infant or an adolescent with a suspected disorder of sex development (Revised 2015). *Clin. Endocrinol.* **2016**, *84*, 771–788. [CrossRef] [PubMed]
24. Fluck, C.; Nordenstrom, A.; Ahmed, S.F.; Ali, S.R.; Berra, M.; Hall, J.; Kohler, B.; Pasterski, V.; Robeva, R.; Schweizer, K.; et al. Standardised data collection for clinical follow-up and assessment of outcomes in differences of sex development (DSD): Recommendations from the COST action DSDnet. *Eur. J. Endocrinol.* **2019**, *181*, 545–564. [CrossRef]
25. Hiort, O.; Birnbaum, W.; Marshall, L.; Wunsch, L.; Werner, R.; Schroder, T.; Dohnert, U.; Holterhus, P.M. Management of disorders of sex development. *Nat. Rev. Endocrinol.* **2014**, *10*, 520–529. [CrossRef]
26. Hiort, O.; Cools, M.; Springer, A.; McElreavey, K.; Greenfield, A.; Wudy, S.A.; Kulle, A.; Ahmed, S.F.; Dessens, A.; Balsamo, A.; et al. Addressing gaps in care of people with conditions affecting sex development and maturation. *Nat. Rev. Endocrinol.* **2019**, *15*, 615–622. [CrossRef]
27. Hutson, J.M.; Grover, S.R.; O'Connell, M.; Pennell, S.D. Malformation syndromes associated with disorders of sex development. *Nat. Rev. Endocrinol.* **2014**, *10*, 476–487. [CrossRef]
28. Cools, M.; Nordenstrom, A.; Robeva, R.; Hall, J.; Westerveld, P.; Fluck, C.; Kohler, B.; Berra, M.; Springer, A.; Schweizer, K.; et al. Caring for individuals with a difference of sex development (DSD): A Consensus Statement. *Nat. Rev. Endocrinol.* **2018**, *14*, 415–429. [CrossRef]
29. van der Straaten, S.; Springer, A.; Zecic, A.; Hebenstreit, D.; Tonnhofer, U.; Gawlik, A.; Baumert, M.; Szeliga, K.; Debulpaep, S.; Desloovere, A.; et al. The External Genitalia Score (EGS): A European Multicenter Validation Study. *J. Clin. Endocrinol. Metab.* **2020**, *105*, e222–e230. [CrossRef]
30. Sathyanarayana, S.; Grady, R.; Redmon, J.B.; Ivicek, K.; Barrett, E.; Janssen, S.; Nguyen, R.; Swan, S.H.; Team, T.S. Anogenital distance and penile width measurements in The Infant Development and the Environment Study (TIDES): Methods and predictors. *J. Pediatr. Urol.* **2015**, *11*, e1-76–e6. [CrossRef]
31. Kulle, A.; Krone, N.; Holterhus, P.M.; Schuler, G.; Greaves, R.F.; Juul, A.; de Rijke, Y.B.; Hartmann, M.F.; Saba, A.; Hiort, O.; et al. Steroid hormone analysis in diagnosis and treatment of DSD: Position paper of EU COST Action BM 1303 'DSDnet'. *Eur. J. Endocrinol.* **2017**, *176*, P1–P9. [CrossRef] [PubMed]
32. Croft, B.; Ayers, K.; Sinclair, A.; Ohnesorg, T. Review disorders of sex development: The evolving role of genomics in diagnosis and gene discovery. *Birth Defects Res. Part C* **2016**, *108*, 337–350. [CrossRef]
33. Audi, L.; Ahmed, S.F.; Krone, N.; Cools, M.; McElreavey, K.; Holterhus, P.M.; Greenfield, A.; Bashamboo, A.; Hiort, O.; Wudy, S.A.; et al. Genetics in Endocrinology: Approaches to molecular genetic diagnosis in the management of differences/disorders of sex development (DSD): Position paper of EU COST Action BM 1303 'DSDnet'. *Eur. J. Endocrinol.* **2018**, *179*, R197–R206. [CrossRef] [PubMed]
34. Avni, F.E.; Lerisson, H.; Lobo, M.L.; Cartigny, M.; Napolitano, M.; Mentzel, H.J.; Riccabona, M.; Wozniak, M.; Kljucevsek, D.; Augdal, T.A.; et al. Plea for a standardized imaging approach to disorders of sex development in neonates: Consensus proposal from European Society of Paediatric Radiology task force. *Pediatr. Radiol.* **2019**, *49*, 1240–1247. [CrossRef] [PubMed]
35. Lindert, J.; Hiort, O.; Tushaus, L.; Tafazzoli-Lari, K.; Wunsch, L. Perineal ultrasound offers useful information in girls with congenital adrenal hyperplasia. *J. Pediatr. Urol.* **2016**, *12*, 427.e1–427.e6. [CrossRef] [PubMed]
36. Marei, M.M.; Fares, A.E.; Abdelsattar, A.H.; Abdullateef, K.S.; Seif, H.; Hassan, M.M.; Elkotby, M.; Eltagy, G.; Elbarbary, M.M. Anatomical measurements of the urogenital sinus in virilized female children due to congenital adrenal hyperplasia. *J. Pediatr. Urol.* **2016**, *12*, 282.e1–282.e8. [CrossRef] [PubMed]
37. Fisher, A.D.; Ristori, J.; Fanni, E.; Castellini, G.; Forti, G.; Maggi, M. Gender identity, gender assignment and reassignment in individuals with disorders of sex development: A major of dilemma. *J. Endocrinol. Investig.* **2016**, *39*, 1207–1224. [CrossRef]
38. Wisniewski, A.B.; Sandberg, D.E. Parenting Children with Disorders of Sex Development (DSD): A Developmental Perspective Beyond Gender. *Horm. Metab. Res.* **2015**, *47*, 375–379. [CrossRef]
39. Wisniewski, A.B.; Tishelman, A.C. Psychological perspectives to early surgery in the management of disorders/differences of sex development. *Curr. Opin. Pediatr.* **2019**, *31*, 570–574. [CrossRef]
40. McCauley, E. Challenges in educating patients and parents about differences in sex development. *Am. J. Med Genet. Part C Semin. Med Genet.* **2017**, *175*, 293–299. [CrossRef]
41. Nordenstrom, A.; Thyen, U. Improving the communication of healthcare professionals with affected children and adolescents. *Endocr. Dev.* **2014**, *27*, 113–127. [CrossRef] [PubMed]
42. Ahmed, S.F.; Khwaja, O.; Hughes, I.A. The role of a clinical score in the assessment of ambiguous genitalia. *Br. J. Urol.* **2000**, *85*, 120–124. [CrossRef] [PubMed]

43. Callens, N.; Kreukels, B.P.C.; van de Grift, T.C. Young Voices: Sexual Health and Transition Care Needs in Adolescents with Intersex/Differences of Sex Development-A Pilot Study. *J. Pediatr. Adolesc. Gynecol.* **2021**, *34*, 176–189. [CrossRef]
44. Crocetti, D.; Monro, S.; Vecchietti, V.; Yeadon-Lee, T. Towards an agency-based model of intersex, variations of sex characteristics (VSC) and DSD/dsd health. *Cult. Health Sex.* **2021**, *23*, 500–515. [CrossRef] [PubMed]
45. Crerand, C.E.; Kapa, H.M.; Litteral, J.L.; Nahata, L.; Combs, B.; Indyk, J.A.; Jayanthi, V.R.; Chan, Y.M.; Tishelman, A.C.; Hansen-Moore, J. Parent perceptions of psychosocial care for children with differences of sex development. *J. Pediatr. Urol.* **2019**, *15*, 522.e1–522.e8. [CrossRef]
46. Sanders, C.; Hall, J.; Sanders, C.; Dessens, A.; Bryce, J.; Callens, N.; Cools, M.; Kourime, M.; Kyriakou, A.; Springer, A.; et al. Involving Individuals with Disorders of Sex Development and Their Parents in Exploring New Models of Shared Learning: Proceedings from a DSDnet COST Action Workshop. *Sex. Dev.* **2018**, *12*, 225–231. [CrossRef]
47. Boyse, K.L.; Gardner, M.; Marvicsin, D.J.; Sandberg, D.E. "It was an overwhelming thing": Parents' needs after infant diagnosis with congenital adrenal hyperplasia. *J. Pediatr. Nurs.* **2014**, *29*, 436–441. [CrossRef]
48. Chawla, R.; Weidler, E.M.; Hernandez, J.; Grimsby, G.; van Leeuwen, K. Utilization of a shared decision-making tool in a female infant with congenital adrenal hyperplasia and genital ambiguity. *J. Pediatr. Endocrinol. Metab.* **2019**, *32*, 643–646. [CrossRef]
49. Siminoff, L.A.; Sandberg, D.E. Promoting Shared Decision Making in Disorders of Sex Development (DSD): Decision Aids and Support Tools. *Horm. Metab. Res.* **2015**, *47*, 335–339. [CrossRef]
50. Karkazis, K.; Tamar-Mattis, A.; Kon, A.A. Genital surgery for disorders of sex development: Implementing a shared decision-making approach. *J. Pediatr. Endocrinol. Metab.* **2010**, *23*, 789–805. [CrossRef]
51. Weidler, E.M.; Baratz, A.; Muscarella, M.; Hernandez, S.J.; van Leeuwen, K. A shared decision-making tool for individuals living with complete androgen insensitivity syndrome. *Semin. Pediatr. Surg.* **2019**, *28*, 150844. [CrossRef] [PubMed]
52. Gesetz zum Schutz von Kindern mit Varianten der Geschlechtsentwicklung. § 1631e BGB. 2021. Available online: https://www.bmj.de/SharedDocs/Gesetzgebungsverfahren/Dokumente/Bgbl_Varianten_der_Geschlechtsentwicklung.pdf;jsessionid=CFCE548CAE6F87495A8485B9E3D8E3B0.1_cid324?__blob=publicationFile&v=3 (accessed on 16 May 2022).
53. Streuli, J.C.; Vayena, E.; Cavicchia-Balmer, Y.; Huber, J. Shaping parents: Impact of contrasting professional counseling on parents' decision making for children with disorders of sex development. *J. Sex. Med.* **2013**, *10*, 1953–1960. [CrossRef] [PubMed]
54. Kranenburg, L.J.C.; Reerds, S.T.H.; Cools, M.; Alderson, J.; Muscarella, M.; Magrite, E.; Kuiper, M.; Abdelgaffar, S.; Balsamo, A.; Brauner, R.; et al. Global Application of the Assessment of Communication Skills of Paediatric Endocrinology Fellows in the Management of Differences in Sex Development Using the ESPE E-Learning.Org Portal. *Horm. Res. Paediatr.* **2017**, *88*, 127–139. [CrossRef] [PubMed]
55. Lampalzer, U.; Briken, P.; Schweizer, K. Dealing With Uncertainty and Lack of Knowledge in Diverse Sex Development: Controversies on Early Surgery and Questions of Consent. *Sex. Med.* **2020**, *8*, 472–489. [CrossRef] [PubMed]

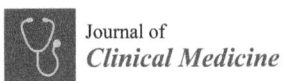

Case Report

Primary Amenorrhea with Apparently Absent Uterus: A Report of Three Cases

Eva Porsius [1,*], Marian Spath [2], Kirsten Kluivers [2], Willemijn Klein [3] and Hedi Claahsen-van der Grinten [1]

1. Department of Pediatric Endocrine Disease, Amalia Children's Hospital, Radboud University Medical Centre, P.O. Box 9101, 6500 HB Nijmegen, The Netherlands; hedi.claahsen@radboudumc.nl
2. Department of Obstetrics and Gynaecology, Radboud University Medical Centre, P.O. Box 9101, 6500 HB Nijmegen, The Netherlands; marian.spath@radboudumc.nl (M.S.); kirsten.kluivers@radboudumc.nl (K.K.)
3. Department of Medical Imaging, Radiology, Radboud University Medical Centre, P.O. Box 9101, 6500 HB Nijmegen, The Netherlands; willemijn.klein@radboudumc.nl
* Correspondence: evaporsius@gmail.com

Abstract: Background: The apparent absence of a uterus upon imaging women with primary amenorrhea appears to lead to a high risk of misdiagnosis, which will lead to significant mental distress in patients. Case: Three young females with primary amenorrhea were referred with a diagnosis of Mayer–Rokitansky–Kuster–Hauser syndrome based on radiological findings of an apparently absent uterus. In two patients, the absence of the uterus could be confirmed, but with various diagnoses. The other patient had a normal but unstimulated uterus due to her hypoestrogenic state. Summary and Conclusion: The presented cases illustrate the broad differential diagnoses and the specific pitfalls of primary amenorrhea with an apparently absent uterus upon imaging. A well-established diagnosis was only possible through a thorough correlation of imaging findings with clinical history, biochemical findings and physical examination.

Keywords: female genital malformations; primary amenorrhea; absent uterus; Müllerian agenesis; DSD

1. Introduction

Primary amenorrhea is a common problem that leads to severe distress in adolescents. Normal puberty starts with breast development at the age of eight to thirteen years. Menarche usually occurs two years after the first signs of puberty, at age eleven to fifteen years. Primary amenorrhea is defined as the absence of menarche by age fifteen or more than three years after the start of breast development [1]. The cause of primary amenorrhea can be due to anatomical abnormalities of the uterus or its outflow tract, and endocrine disorders of the gonads, pituitary gland or hypothalamus [2,3]. The presence or absence of a uterus can help to categorize primary amenorrhea, as illustrated in Figure 1.

Uterus absence in otherwise healthy females with normal external genitalia can be caused by different conditions within differences in sex development (DSD) conditions. Therefore, a DSD condition, such as Müllerian agenesis, testosterone synthesis defect or complete androgen insensitivity syndrome (CAIS), should be considered as the underlying cause of primary amenorrhea.

Pelvic ultrasound and magnetic resonance imaging (MRI) are good methods to visualize Müllerian structures [3,4]. When the uterus cannot be detected by ultrasound, MRI is advised for detailed imaging of Müllerian structures, ovaries, the vagina and kidneys [3]. It has to be considered that, especially in prepubertal state, a present uterus may remain undetected, since in the hypoestrogenic state the uterus is small and not easy to visualize. The interpretation of imaging findings by an experienced radiologist with knowledge of the normal appearance of the uterus and ovaries during different phases of growth and development is therefore preferred [4].

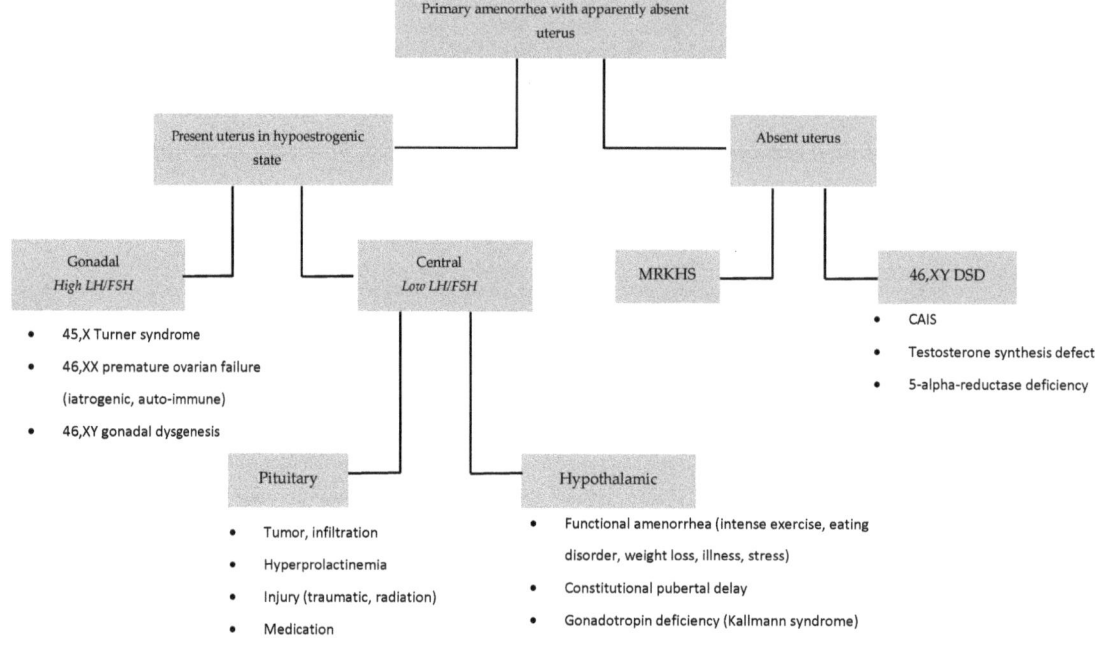

Figure 1. Differential diagnoses of primary amenorrhea with apparently absent uterus on imaging in women with normal external genitalia. LH: luteinizing hormone; FSH: follicle-stimulating hormone; MRKHS: Mayer–Rokitansky–Küster–Hauser syndrome; DSD: differences in sex development; CAIS: complete androgen insensitivity syndrome.

In this paper, we present three cases of young women who were referred to our hospital presenting with primary amenorrhea and an apparently absent uterus. Our aim is to point out the importance of correlating imaging findings with clinical history, biochemical findings and physical examination, and provide guidance for distinguishing the various diagnoses of primary amenorrhea with an absent uterus upon imaging. This is important because these cases are rare, but various medical practitioners could encounter them and misdiagnosis will lead to significant mental distress in patients.

2. Case 1

A seventeen-year-old girl was referred to the local gynecologist because of primary amenorrhea. Puberty had started with breast development and pubarche at the age of ten. She had used the oral contraceptive pill, but no withdrawal bleeding ever occurred. According to the patient, penetration during sexual intercourse was possible without pain. However, from a physical examination and vaginal ultrasound, a short and blind-ending vagina was found. The MRI suggested an absent uterus, normally located ovaries and normal kidneys (Figure 2). With the suspicion of Mayer–Rokitansky–Küster–Hauser syndrome (MRKHS), the patient was referred to our expert center. An MRI demonstrated no vaginal, myometrial or cervical tissue, with some fibrous and lipomatous tissue at this location. The ovaries had normal cystic appearance and were situated in the broad ligament. Karyotype was 46,XX. A hormonal examination showed normal endocrine parameters (Table 1). With these results, a diagnosis of MRKHS was confirmed and the patient received information about the etiology and consequences of this diagnosis.

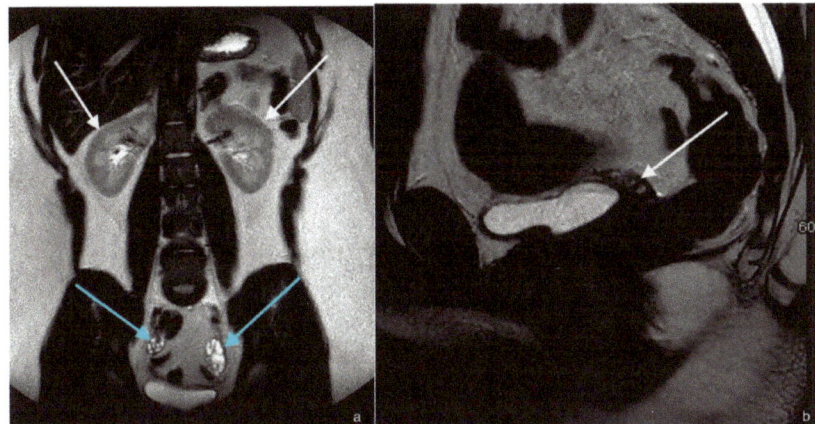

Figure 2. Case 1. (**a**) Coronal T2-weighted image of the abdomen, showing two normal kidneys (white arrows) as well as two normal ovaries (blue arrows). (**b**) Mid-sagittal T2-weighted image of the pelvis, demonstrating a triangular shape between bladder and rectum, which is the fibro-adipose remnant tissue of the aplastic uterus, without any endometrial or myometrial organization (white arrow).

Table 1. Overview of important findings in three cases with primary amenorrhea, based on Mayer–Rokitansky–Küster–Hauser syndrome (MRKHS), complete androgen insensitivity syndrome (CAIS) and hypogonadotropic hypogonadism of unknown origin.

		Case 1	Case 2	Case 3
	Diagnosis	MRKHS	CAIS	Hypogonadotropic hypogonadism e.c.i.
	History	Normal start of breast development and pubarche	Normal start of breast development, no pubarche	Delayed and incomplete breast development, normal pubarche
	Physical examination	Tanner M4 P4 Female external genitalia with no virilization Short blind-ending vagina	Tanner M5 P1 Female external genitalia with no virilization. Tall stature. No axillary hair	Tanner M1-2 P2-3 Female external genitalia with no virilization BMI 15.8 kg/m^2 (−2.2 SD) Height 1.56 m (−1.78 SD)
Biochemical analysis	reference values			
LH	2.4–12.6 E/L (follicular), 14.0–95.6 (ovular), 1.0–11.4 (luteal)	38.8	24	0.5
FSH	3.5–12.5 E/L (follicular); 4.7–21.5 (ovular); 1.7–7.7 (luteal)	6.6	2.8	1.2
Estradiol	45–854 pmol/L (follicular); 151–1461 (ovular); 82–1251 (luteal)	470	78	<18
AMH	0.52–12.01 ug/L	2.5	1292	10.1
Testosterone	0.52–2.0 nmol/L		13	

Table 1. Cont.

		Case 1	Case 2	Case 3
Progesterone	<1.3 (follicular); 1.3–12 (mid cycle); 19–120 (luteal) nmol/L	1.7	<0.25	
Prolactin	100–760 mE/L			250
TSH	0.27–4.20 mE/L			2.5
	Karyotype	46,XX	46,XY	46,XX
Imaging findings	ultrasound	No visualization of uterus or ovaries	No visualization of uterus or ovaries	No visualization of uterus or ovaries
	MRI report on primary investigation	Absent uterus, impression of hypoplastic vagina. Normal multicystic ovaries	Absent uterus and presence of a short vagina. Normal ovaries	Normal multicystic ovaries and a small uterus of 2.3 × 1.3 cm, described as rudimentary uterus
	MRI after referral	Lipofibromatous tissue at location of the uterus, no endo- myometrial or cervical structures. Normal multicystic ovaries	Underdeveloped Müllerian structures. Gonads with (ovo)testicular aspect	Small uterus with normal endo- and myometrial tissue, normal multicystic ovaries

BMI: body mass index; SD: standard deviation; MRI: magnetic resonance imaging; LH: luteinizing hormone; FSH: follicle-stimulating hormone; AMH: anti-Müllerian hormone; TSH: thyroid-stimulating hormone.

3. Case 2

A seventeen-year-old girl presented with primary amenorrhea after a normal start to puberty. Breast development started at the age of twelve years and she had a growth spurt two years later. The physical examination showed the normal anatomy of the vulva and shaved pubic hair, and the vaginal depth upon digital palpation was 3–4 cm (reference 7–15 cm [5]). The uterus and ovaries could not be visualized by pelvic ultrasound (Figure 3a). MRI performed in the local hospital confirmed the absence of a normal uterus and presence of a short vagina. In this MRI report, normal ovaries were described. These results lead to the assumption of an MRKHS diagnosis. This was explained to the patient and vaginal dilation therapy was suggested.

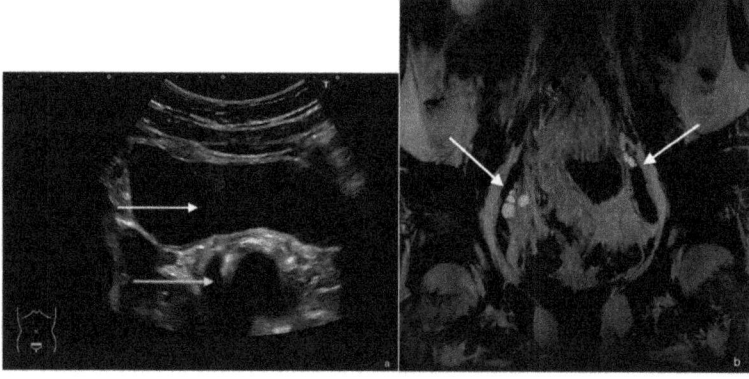

Figure 3. Case 2. (**a**) Ultrasound of the pelvis, demonstrating the rectum (blue arrow) direct dorsal to the bladder (white arrow), without uterus in between. (**b**) Coronal T2-weighted MR image of the pelvis, with the white arrows indicating the gonads with partially solid tissue and partially cystic, a suspected aspect of ovotestes.

She was referred to our expert center with suspicion of MRKHS. In the physical exam, we noted her tall stature (height +1.17 SDS) and very sparse axillary and pubic hair. After the specialized radiologist reviewed the MRI, the previously described ovaries actually appeared as atypical gonadal structures with a large solid part, suspected of being (ovo)testicular tissue (Figure 3b). A hormonal examination showed high levels of anti-Müllerian hormone (AMH) and testosterone (Table 1). Genetic diagnostics confirmed the suspicion of a 46,XY karyotype and an androgen receptor gene mutation (hemizygous variant NM_000044.2(AR):c.2594A>T, p.(Asp865Val)), confirming the diagnosis of CAIS. Follow up by our DSD team is continued to guide her during vaginal dilation therapy, offer psychological support and screening for a possible malignant transformation of the abdominal testes.

4. Case 3

A sixteen-year-old girl presented with delayed puberty and primary amenorrhea. Breast development started at age fourteen, but no further progression occurred after tanner stages 1–2. Axillary and pubic hair also developed up to tanner stage 2. There were no signs of virilization. She had a short stature and low weight (Table 1). Bone age was delayed 3 years according to Gruelich and Pyle using the automatic BoneXpert method [6]. There were no signs of eating disorders, malabsorption or other chronic illness. The mother had normal puberty with menarche at twelve years old. The father experienced late but spontaneous puberty. There was no history of medication use, except sporadic corticosteroid ointment for eczema. Hormonal serum analysis showed low FSH, LH and estradiol levels, normal thyroid function and prolactin levels (Table 1). The karyotype was 46,XX. Abdominal ultrasound performed at the local hospital showed no uterus or ovaries. Subsequent MRI showed normal ovaries and a small uterus (2.3 × 1.3 cm), described as a rudimentary uterus suspected for MRKHS.

She was referred to our expert center with a diagnosis of MRKHS. Ultrasound and MRI revision by our radiologist showed a small uterus with visible myo- and endometrial tissue, which was interpreted as an unstimulated hypoestrogenic uterus (Figure 4). A further diagnostic evaluation of the etiology of hypogonadotropic hypogonadism was performed. Cerebral MRI showed no pathology in the hypothalamus or pituitary gland. Exome sequencing known genes connected to hypogonadotropic hypogonadism showed no mutations. Pubertal induction with estrogen therapy was started, which resulted in breast development, endometrial thickening and menarche.

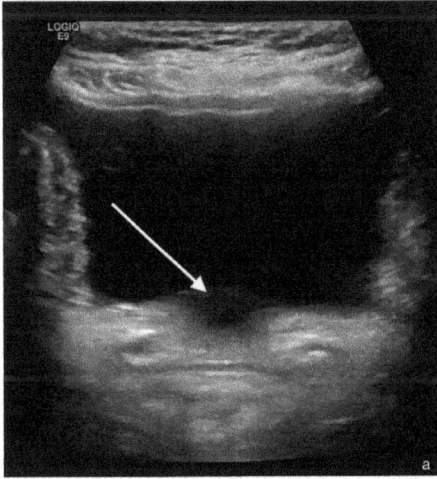
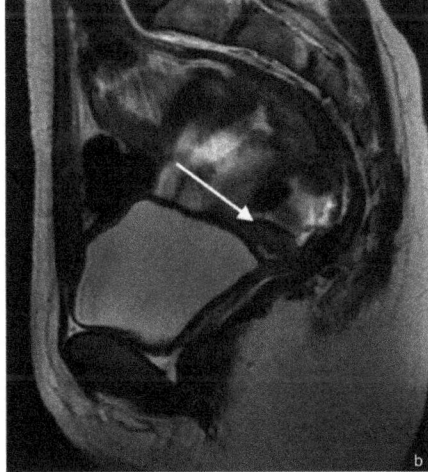

Figure 4. *Cont.*

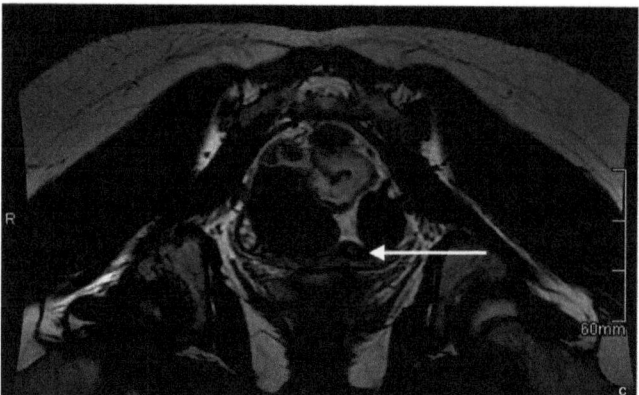

Figure 4. Case 3. (**a**) Ultrasound of the pelvis. The white arrow indicates a small uterus behind the bladder. (**b**). Mid-sagittal T2-weighted MR image, demonstrating a small uterus (white arrow). (**c**) The oblique-coronal T2-weighted images demonstrate clearly that there is an architecture of endometrial and myometrial tissue (white arrow).

5. Discussion

This study presents three patients with primary amenorrhea, who were referred to our expert clinic with a (mis)diagnosis of MRKHS because of radiological findings of an apparently absent uterus. In two patients, the absence of the uterus could be confirmed, but with various diagnoses (MRKHS resp. CAIS). The other patient had a normal but unstimulated uterus. Our case report shows that the apparent absence of a uterus upon imaging in women with primary amenorrhea appears to lead to a high risk of misdiagnosis. The presented cases illustrate the broad range of diagnoses of primary amenorrhea and specific pitfalls. A well-established diagnosis was only possible through considering the combination of clinical history, physical examination, biochemical evaluation and assessment of imaging by an experienced radiologist.

During the prenatal development of 46,XX individuals, the Müllerian ducts fuse in absence of AMH to form the uterovaginal canal. In syndromes with Müllerian agenesis, such as MRKHS, this process fails, resulting in the absence of the uterus and upper part of the vagina [7]. In 46,XY individuals, AMH stimulates the regression of Müllerian ducts, resulting in absence of the uterus. Testosterone and dihydrotestosterone are responsible for the virilization of external genitalia. The effect of these androgens is compromised in androgen receptor defects and testosterone synthesis or metabolizing defects. A 46,XY female with CAIS but normal functioning AMH will thereby have external female features in the absence of a uterus and will have testes instead of ovaries [8].

The first step in the evaluation of primary amenorrhea is carefully looking through clinical history and physical examination. Women with MRKHS experience a normal start of puberty with age-appropriate breast development and pubarche, but primary amenorrhea as an isolated symptom [7]. In CAIS, there is a normal onset of breast development, but no or very sparse axillary and pubic hair. A Tanner stage examination is important since patients will often unknowingly misinterpret pubarche. Height is taller than general. Acne and sweat odor are absent. Breasts and female adiposity can develop through the action of estradiol deriving from the peripheral aromatization of testosterone [8]. Delayed pubertal development in 46,XX individuals with an absence of breast development and menarche is caused by estrogen absence, due to ovarian or pituitary/hypothalamic causes.

Thus, assessing patient history and physical findings carefully an accurate diagnosis can be made. However, as the impact of these diagnoses is great, biochemical analysis, imaging or karyotype analysis is conducted to support this. A careful consideration of necessary diagnostics will prevent misinterpretation and misdiagnosis.

LH, FSH, progesterone, estradiol, TSH and prolactin can guide in finding possible endocrine causes of primary amenorrhea [2]. In response to our cases, we suggest adding AMH and testosterone to give direction in determining possible 46,XY DSD conditions. Karyotype analysis should always be performed when 46,XY DSD conditions are considered.

In women with normal secondary sexual characteristics but primary amenorrhea, pelvic ultrasound is advised to search for possible anatomical causes [2,3]. In case of an apparently absent uterus on ultrasound, we advise performing MRI and consulting a specialized radiologist. In CAIS patients, no Müllerian structures will be found and gonadal tissue might be testicular or maldifferentiated. In women with an absent uterus because of MRKHS, absence might not always be a full absence. Wang et al. [9] described bilateral Müllerian rudiments seen on MRI in 95% of MRKHS women and normally located ovaries in 68.7%. The Müllerian rudiments are generally small with only one-layer differentiation. There is also a high incidence of renal (~30%) and skeletal (~10–40%) anomalies [7].

In women with delayed breast development, uterus imaging is not advised, since mostly estrogen deficiency will be the cause of primary amenorrhea. An important consideration is that, in the hypoestrogenic state, the uterus is small and unstimulated and can therefore be difficult to visualize. Berglund et al. [10] described the association of an apparently absent uterus with primary ovarian insufficiency in their review of the literature. Estrogen deficiency has previously resulted in misdiagnosis as MRKHS in 22/25 patients (88%) with primary ovarian insufficiency. Michala et al. [11] demonstrates this as well in their description of ten patients with misdiagnoses of uterine agenesis based on imaging and laparoscopic findings. They suggest that imaging should be undertaken by clinicians with experience in management of this age group and in some girls it may be necessary to delay final diagnosis until after puberty or the administration of estrogen therapy.

In case of absent uterus upon imaging, a progestin challenge test [3] will probably not lead to vaginal bleeding. In modern practice, there seems to be no additional value for this test, but a high risk of further delay of correct diagnosis.

The diagnosis of an absent uterus and vagina leads to a negative impact on the affected women's level of psychological distress and self-esteem [12]. Additionally, these women are confronted with sexuality and fertility issues at a young age. In the case of the misdiagnosis of MRKHS instead of CAIS, the adolescent will be confronted with confusing information: first the absence of uterus and vagina and subsequent information on afunctional gonads. This has even further fertility consequences and, therefore, it is important to make an early correct diagnosis. Confirmation by a DSD team is advised [3]. This specialized team consists of a gynecologist, endocrinologist, radiologist, psychologist, geneticist, urologist and sexologist.

6. Conclusions

The presented cases illustrate the broad differential diagnosis and the specific pitfalls of primary amenorrhea with an apparently absent uterus upon imaging. It is important not to draw premature conclusions from findings of an apparently absent uterus from imaging alone. A well-established diagnosis was only possible with a thorough correlation of imaging findings with clinical history, biochemical findings and physical examination.

Author Contributions: E.P. and H.C.-v.d.G. participated in the design and planning of the article. E.P. performed data collection and drafted the manuscript. K.K., M.S., W.K. and H.C.-v.d.G. revised the manuscript critically. All authors have read and agreed to the published version of the manuscript.

Funding: This research received no external funding.

Institutional Review Board Statement: Ethical review and approval were waived for this study due to the rules of our hospitals Research Ethics Committee. Retrospective research with patient files, where the patients are not physically involved in the research and the data were collected primarily for patients care and not primarily for research purposes, is not considered to be subject to the Medical Research Involving Human Subjects Act.

Informed Consent Statement: Written permission to report these cases was obtained from all patients. No ethics committee or institutional review board approval was required, according to the local Research Ethics Committee.

Data Availability Statement: Not applicable.

Acknowledgments: We would like to thank our patients for their permission to use their history and clinical data.

Conflicts of Interest: The authors declare no conflict of interest.

References

1. Teede, H.J.; Misso, M.L.; Costello, M.F.; Dokras, A.; Laven, J.; Moran, L.; Piltonen, T.; Norman, R.J.; International, P.N. Recommendations from the international evidence-based guideline for the assessment and management of polycystic ovary syndrome. *Clin. Endocrinol.* **2018**, *89*, 251–268. [CrossRef] [PubMed]
2. Klein, D.A.; Poth, M.A. Amenorrhea: An approach to diagnosis and management. *Am. Fam. Physician* **2013**, *87*, 781–788. [PubMed]
3. Nederlandse Vereniging Obstetrie & Gynaecologie (NVOG). Primaire Amenorroe. Available online: https://richtlijnendatabase.nl/richtlijn/primaire_amenorroe/primaire_amenorroe_-_startpagina.html (accessed on 5 May 2022).
4. Rosenberg, H.K. Sonography of the pelvis in patients with primary amenorrhea. *Endocrinol. Metab. Clin. N. Am.* **2009**, *38*, 739–760. [CrossRef] [PubMed]
5. Pendergrass, P.B.; Reeves, C.A.; Belovicz, M.W.; Molter, D.J.; White, J.H. The shape and dimensions of the human vagina as seen in three-dimensional vinyl polysiloxane casts. *Gynecol. Obstet. Investig.* **1996**, *42*, 178–182. [CrossRef] [PubMed]
6. van Rijn, R.R.; Lequin, M.H.; Thodberg, H.H. Automatic determination of Greulich and Pyle bone age in healthy Dutch children. *Pediatr. Radiol.* **2009**, *39*, 591–597. [CrossRef] [PubMed]
7. Herlin, M.K.; Petersen, M.B.; Brannstrom, M. Mayer-Rokitansky-Kuster-Hauser (MRKH) syndrome: A comprehensive update. *Orphanet J. Rare Dis.* **2020**, *15*, 214. [CrossRef] [PubMed]
8. Lanciotti, L.; Cofini, M.; Leonardi, A.; Bertozzi, M.; Penta, L.; Esposito, S. Different Clinical Presentations and Management in Complete Androgen Insensitivity Syndrome (CAIS). *Int. J. Environ. Res. Public Health* **2019**, *16*, 1268. [CrossRef] [PubMed]
9. Wang, Y.; He, Y.L.; Yuan, L.; Yu, J.C.; Xue, H.D.; Jin, Z.Y. Typical and atypical pelvic MRI characteristics of Mayer-Rokitansky-Kuster-Hauser syndrome: A comprehensive analysis of 201 patients. *Eur. Radiol.* **2020**, *30*, 4014–4022. [CrossRef] [PubMed]
10. Berglund, A.; Burt, E.; Cameron-Pimblett, A.; Davies, M.C.; Conway, G.S. A critical assessment of case reports describing absent uterus in subjects with oestrogen deficiency. *Clin. Endocrinol.* **2019**, *90*, 822–826. [CrossRef] [PubMed]
11. Michala, L.; Aslam, N.; Conway, G.S.; Creighton, S.M. The clandestine uterus: Or how the uterus escapes detection prior to puberty. *BJOG* **2010**, *117*, 212–215. [CrossRef] [PubMed]
12. Heller-Boersma, J.G.; Schmidt, U.H.; Edmonds, D.K. Psychological distress in women with uterovaginal agenesis (Mayer-Rokitansky-Kuster-Hauser Syndrome, MRKH). *Psychosomatics* **2009**, *50*, 277–281. [CrossRef] [PubMed]

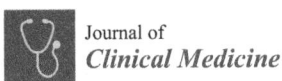

Case Report

Ectopic Prostate Tissue in the Uterine Cervix of a Female with Non-Classic Congenital Adrenal Hyperplasia—A Case Report

Lea Tschaidse [1], Matthias K. Auer [1], Ilja Dubinski [2], Christian Lottspeich [1], Hanna Nowotny [1], Heinrich Schmidt [2], Nadezda Gut [3] and Nicole Reisch [1,*]

[1] Medizinische Klinik und Poliklinik IV, Klinikum der Universität München, LMU München, 80336 Munich, Germany; lea.tschaidse@med.uni-muenchen.de (L.T.); matthias.auer@med.uni-muenchen.de (M.K.A.); christian.lottspeich@med.uni-muenchen.de (C.L.); hanna.nowotny@med.uni-muenchen.de (H.N.)

[2] Department of Pediatric Endocrinology, Dr. von Haunersches Children's Hospital, Klinikum der Universität München, LMU München, 80336 Munich, Germany; ilja.dubinski@med.uni-muenchen.de (I.D.); heinrich.schmidt@med.uni-muenchen.de (H.S.)

[3] Zentrum für Pathologie Allgäu (ZfPA), Medizinisches Versorgungzentrum am Klinikum Kempten, 87439 Kempten, Germany; dr.n.gut@googlemail.com

* Correspondence: nicole.reisch@med.uni-muenchen.de

Abstract: Introduction: The occurrence of ectopic prostate tissue in the female genital tract is rare and has only been described sporadically. The origin of these lesions is unclear, but their appearance seems to be associated with various forms of androgen excess, including androgen therapy for transgender treatment or disorders of sex development, such as classic congenital adrenal hyperplasia (CAH). This is the first described case of ectopic prostate tissue in the cervix uteri of a 46,XX patient with a confirmed diagnosis of non-classic CAH due to 21-OHD and a history of mild adrenal androgen excess. Case presentation: We describe a 34-year-old patient with a genetic diagnosis of non-classic CAH due to 21-hydroxylase deficiency (21-OHD) with a female karyo- and phenotype and a history of mild adrenal androgen excess. Due to dysplasia in the cervical smear, conization had to be performed, revealing ectopic prostate tissue in the cervix uteri of the patient. Conclusions: An association between androgen excess and the occurrence of prostate tissue is likely and should therefore be considered as a differential diagnosis for atypical tissue in the female genital tract.

Keywords: 21-hydroxylase deficiency; androgen excess; virilization; ectopic prostate tissue; hyperandrogenemia

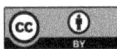

1. Background

There have been several reports of prostate tissue or even whole prostate glands in the female genital tract [1–5]. The cause of the development of this tissue is still unclear, since prostatic tissue in women without a history of hormonal, gonadal or genetic disorders has been reported as a very rare incidental finding [2]. Nevertheless, its appearance seems to be influenced by increased androgen concentrations, as several reports show the occurrence of prostatic tissue in the vaginal specimens of patients with different disorders of sexual development (DSD) associated with androgen excess [1,3–5] and in 46,XX patients who underwent testosterone therapy due to gender dysphoria [1].

Congenital adrenal hyperplasia due to 21-hydroxylase deficiency (CAH 21-OHD) is an autosomal recessive disorder and one of the most common forms of DSD [6]. It is characterized by cortisol deficiency and an adrenocorticotropic hormone (ACTH)-driven adrenal androgen excess [7]. Based on the clinical manifestation, CAH can be divided into classic, with or without salt wasting, or the non-classic form [8]. With a frequency of about 1:15,000 [8,9], classic CAH is the rarer but much more severe form and is usually diagnosed at birth or during infancy. Due to severe cortisol and possible aldosterone deficiency, the classic form of CAH is a life-threatening disease, making lifelong therapy necessary. Additionally, androgen excess during embryonic development leads to prenatal virilization of the external genitalia in 46,XX patients with classic CAH. The development of internal genital organs is unaffected, as this is determined by genetic sex [7].

The non-classic form, on the other hand, represents the mild variant of the disease and is much more common than classic CAH, with a frequency of 1:200 to 1:1000 [9,10]. Affected patients have sufficient cortisol synthesis and typically develop symptoms of mild androgen excess around the age of puberty, such as acne, hirsutism, alopecia, menstrual irregularities or an unfulfilled desire to have children. The development of external genitalia is normal [11].

In this report, we describe the first case of a patient with a confirmed diagnosis of non-classic CAH due to 21-OHD with a female karyo- and phenotype and ectopic prostate tissue in the cervix uteri. A timeline of the patient's medical history and care is described in Table 1. Written informed consent was obtained from the patient before submission and publication of this case report. This work was conducted in accordance with the Declaration of Helsinki, and the protocol was approved by the Ethics Committee of the Medical Faculty of Ludwig Maximilians University Munich (Project number 19-558).

Table 1. Timeline of patient's medical history.

Patient Visits	Patient Age	Clinical Presentation	Diagnostic Findings	Consequences and Procedure
Visit 1 10/1997	10	- Advanced bone age - Pubes: Tanner Stage V - Breast development: Tanner Stage V - Menarche at 10 - Mild acne - Normal external genitalia	- Premature development - Hyperandrogenaemia and elevated 17-OHP in serum - Genetic confirmation of non-classic CAH (compound heterozygous I2G/P30L)	- Starting hydrocortisone therapy 20 mg/day
Visit 2 05/2000	12	- Normal external genitalia - Mild acne - Regular cycle	- Hyperandrogenaemia and elevated 17-OHP level in serum - Elevated pregnanetriol in a 24-h urine sample	- Continuation of hydrocortisone therapy with 20 mg/day
Visit 3 07/2006	18	- No Acne - Mild clitoral hypertrophy	- Hyperandrogenaemia and elevated 17-OHP level in serum	- No therapy at patient's request
Visit 4 05/2016	28	- Hirsutism - Regular cycle	- Hyperandrogenaemia and elevated 17-OHP level in serum	- Starting prednisolone therapy with 2 mg/day to achieve pregnancy
Visit 5 10/2021	34	- Hirsutism - Scarring acne	- Hyperandrogenaemia and elevated 17-OHP level in serum - Pathological cervical smear: (HPV)-positive dysplasia	- Scheduling a conization
Visit 6 01/2022 Post-conzation follow-up	34	- Hirsutism - Scarring acne	- Hyperandrogenaemia and elevated 17-OHP level in serum - Ectopic, metaplastic prostatic tissue in the cervix uteri (resected in total)	- Starting therapy with modified release hydrocortisone 10mg/day and an anti-androgenic oral contraceptive

Depicted is the patients' medical history with clinical and diagnostic findings at each visit at our clinic, as well as treatment and further procedure. 17-OHP 17-Hydroxyprogesterone A4 Androstenedione DHEA-S Dehydroepiandrosterone sulfate.

2. Patient Information

We report on a 34-year-old patient who has been under irregular care of our pediatric and adult endocrinology departments for years due to non-classic CAH. The diagnosis of non-classic CAH was made due to premature development and biochemical presentation. The patient presented to our pediatric clinic for the first time at the age of 10, with an advanced bone age of 14 years, with pubes and breast development on both sides documented as Tanner Stage V and with menarche at the age of 10. Biochemically, the patient showed elevated 17-hydroxyprogesterone (17-OHP) concentrations and hyperandrogenemia with elevated androstenedione (A4), dehydroepiandrosterone-sulfate (DHEA-S) and testosterone concentrations (Table 1; Figure 1). The diagnosis of non-classic CAH was confirmed by genetic testing, showing a compound heterozygous mutation with I2G and P30L mutations. This genotype is traditionally associated with non-classic CAH, but phenotypes may vary [12]. Adrenal insufficiency was excluded. Although the patient had received hydrocortisone therapy with 20 mg hydrocortisone per day between the ages of 10 and 14 years to suppress adrenal androgen synthesis, she continued to demonstrate inadequate hormonal control, as shown in Table 1 and Figure 1. At the patient's request, hydrocortisone therapy ended after body growth was completed, with a final height of 160.4 cm at the age of 14 years. The patient gave birth to two healthy children at the ages of 27 and 31 years after receiving infertility treatment with clomiphene and under a temporary intake of prednisolone, respectively. After conception of the second pregnancy, the intake of prednisolone was terminated by the patient.

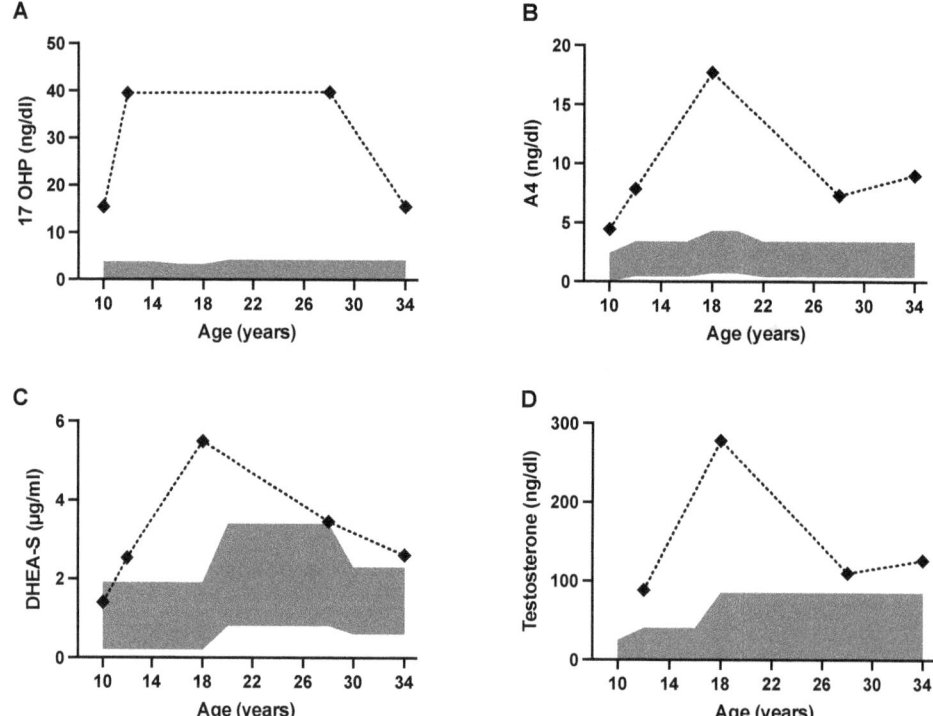

Figure 1. 17-OHP and androgen levels of the patients at different ages.

Graphical representation of increased 17-OHP and androgen levels of the patient at different ages, depicted as black data points in relation to sex- and age-specific reference range, shown as a gray area. 17-OHP 17-Hydroxyprogesterone A4 Androstenedione DHEA-S Dehydroepiandrosterone sulfate.

3. Clinical Findings

On occasional visits to our clinic, the patient continued to show clinical signs of hyperandrogenemia, such as scarring acne of the upper body and both upper arms, mild hirsutism of the face and mild clitoral hypertrophy. Still, the patient did not wish to receive medication on a regular basis.

4. Diagnostic Assessment

At each visit, our patient showed biochemical hyperandrogenemia, documented as the laboratory findings of an untreated, non-classical CAH, with elevated 17-OHP, A4, DHEA-S and testosterone concentrations.

Cervical smears were taken regularly as part of the gynecological check-ups. Recently, a cervical smear revealed an abnormal result with human papillomavirus (HPV)-positive dysplasia. Therefore, conization had to be performed.

5. Therapeutic Intervention and Follow-Up

The examination of the portioconisate confirmed a high-grade squamous intraepithelial lesion, as already found in the previously performed cervical smear. However, atypical tissue in the cervix was detected in one quadrant of the conisate. Hematoxylin and eosin (HE) staining showed a normal transition from ecto- to endocervix in most of the specimens, with unremarkable squamous epithelium as well as mucinous epithelium on the surface and in the glands, as depicted in Figure 2A. The atypical metaplastic tissue appeared to be of glandular origin, as depicted in Figure 2A in the HE staining. The atypical glandular proliferations in the endocervix showed the typical morphology of the prostate glands, not the glands of the endocervix. Metaplastic prostate tissue was located outside the endocervical glandular field. The glands showed diffuse positivity for prostate-specific antigen (PSA) and NKX3.1, as depicted in Figure 2C,D. Further immunohistochemical examination of the area showed no expression of p16 and the proliferation rate with Ki 67 was not found to be increased. The morphology of the tissue section and findings on immunohistochemistry support the presence of ectopic, metaplastic prostatic tissue in the cervix uteri, which was resected in total. A subsequent analysis showed a PSA level of 0.013 ng/dL in our patient before conization, which dropped to 0.007 ng/dL afterwards.

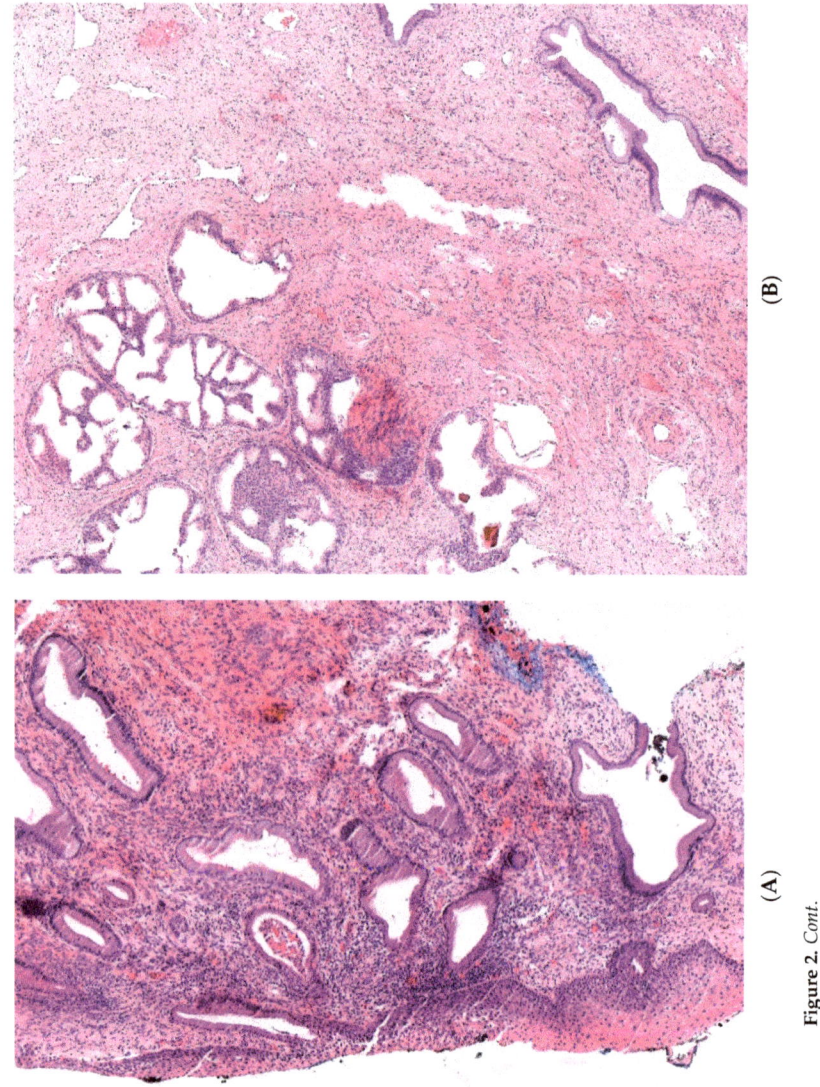

Figure 2. Cont.

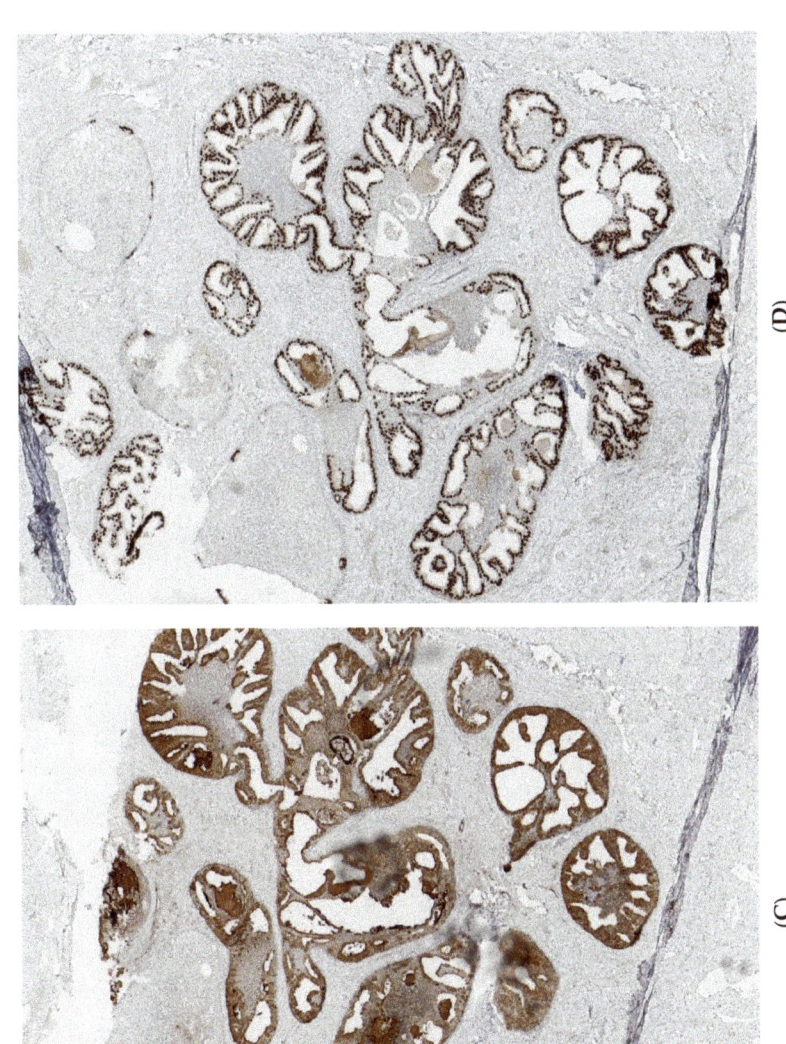

Figure 2. Histological features of cervix tissue in HE staining with normal ecto- and endocervix in most specimens (**A**). Histologic features of ectopic prostate tissue with gland ducts in HE staining (**B**) and diffuse positivity in immunohistochemical testing with PSA (**C**) and NKX3.1 (**D**).

6. Discussion

The cell morphology, as well as the positivity for PSA and NKX3.1 of the atypical tissue sections found in the patient, is consistent with previous publications on prostate tissue [1,2].

Most reported cases of ectopic prostatic tissue in females are related to a history of severe androgen excess. In particular, several reports of prostate tissue in patients with DSD have been published. Anderson et al. [1] found prostatic tissue in vaginal specimens of multiple patients, one of which likely presented with partial androgen insensitivity due to 46,XY DSD, another with ovotesticular disorder of differentiation and of patients with classic congenital adrenal hyperplasia (46,XX). In 46,XX patients with classic CAH and a male phenotype due to delayed diagnosis, fully developed prostate glands have also been reported [4,5,13–15]. Wesselius et al. [3] even described a case of prostate cancer in such a patient, although to our knowledge, this is the only reported case of this kind. However, our patient had only a mild, non-classic form of CAH.

Single cases of prostatic tissue in the female genital tract have even been described in very few patients without any clinical record of hormonal, gonadal or genetic alterations affecting androgen synthesis or effect. McCluggage et al. [2] found ectopic prostate tissue in the lower female genital tract of women who had undergone loop excision due to an abnormal cervical smear. They [2] and others [16] also found ectopic prostate tissue in the cervix uteri. The origin of this prostate tissue is still unknown, but theories of metaplasia and developmental abnormalities have been discussed [16]. Prostate tissue develops from the periurethral glands that occur during early embryonic development in both females and males. Sustained androgen stimulation in males causes these glands to proliferate, whereas in females, they regress due to a lack of stimulus [16,17]. In line, a common feature of the cases described in the literature is elevated androgen levels over a long period of time, either due to increased endogenous androgens [1,4,5] or due to testosterone therapy, e.g., for transgender treatment [1]. Furthermore, the induction of prostatic metaplasia in vaginal tissue through androgens in animal models has been shown [18]. This hypothesis is also supported by the reports of Anderson et al. [1] and Singh et al. [19], in which prostate tissue was found in the lower genital tract of 46,XX patients after having received high-dose testosterone therapy due to gender dysphoria. It has even been suggested that prolonged androgen exposure results in more mature, further differentiated prostate cells [1]. As our patient refused treatment for most of her life, mildly elevated androgen concentrations were likely potential influencing factors in this case. In addition, hyperandrogenaemia continued to be evident during the short time she was receiving drug therapy (Table 1). The location of the tissue in our patient, namely at the cervix uteri, would fit the theory of developmental anomaly. Since the uterus and the urogenital sinus are in close proximity during embryonic development, there could be scattering of the periurethral glands, which could later present as prostatic tissue [16].

Since PSA can sometimes be detected in 46,XX patients with classic CAH [5,20,21] and elevated PSA levels have been described in 46,XX patients with classic CAH and prostate cancer [3,17], we subsequently determined the PSA level from samples before conization and thus removal of prostate tissue in our patient. The PSA level was below the male reference value (<0.03 ng/mL), most likely due to the small amount of ectopic tissue. Nevertheless, PSA should not be underestimated as a biomarker since Paulino Mda et al. [20] found good specificity and sensitivity of PSA for prostatic tissue in girls with classic CAH.

Thus far, prostate tissue has almost exclusively been reported in patients with classic CAH, who—in periods of poor disease control—are exposed to substantially higher androgen concentrations [3–5,13–15,17,20–24], but not in non-classic CAH. In a study by Paulino Mda et al. [20] prostatic tissue could be detected in five out of 32 girls with classic CAH through MRI, which indicates a prevalence of 15.6% in classic CAH. The number of unknown cases may therefore be significantly higher, as small scattered tissue sections could not be detected through this method. Anderson et al. [1] also described prostate tissue only in the urogenital tract of patients with classic CAH but not of non-classic CAH.

The discrepancy between the reported frequency in classic and non-classic CAH could be due to the actual increased occurrence of this tissue in patients with classic CAH or due to selection bias. Since female patients with non-classic CAH do not present with prenatal virilization of the external genitalia, there is no need for genital reconstruction, making surgically removed tissue from these patients for examination hardly available.

To our knowledge, there is only one case report of a 46,XX patient with alleged non-classic CAH and prostate tissue found in the vaginal tissue and cervix uteri by Kim, Park [25]. The female patient presented in young adulthood with an expressed desire for gender reassignment due to a male gender identity. She showed significant clinical virilisation, such as hirsutism, steroid acne, primary amenorrhea and an elongated clitoris of 5 cm. A diagnosis of non-classic CAH was made based on the clinical presentation and one-time elevated laboratory values of ACTH, adrenal androgens and 17-OHP. There was no confirmation of the diagnosis by a short synacthen test or genetic testing [25]. However, given that the patient showed substantial virilization of the external genitalia and highly elevated basal 17-OHP (130 ng/mL), the diagnosis of non-classic CAH is unlikely, but rather classic simple virilizing CAH with presumable higher concentrations of adrenal androgens was the case. Interestingly, other developmental remnants, such as ovarian and testicular adrenal rests, are common in poorly controlled patients with classic CAH due to elevated concentrations of adrenocorticotropic hormones. However, in non-classic CAH, most likely due to only mild hormonal changes, these remnants have not been described.

Thus, to our knowledge, this is the first described case of ectopic prostate tissue in the cervix uteri of a 46,XX patient with a confirmed diagnosis of non-classic CAH due to 21-OHD and a history of mild adrenal androgen excess. As ectopic prostatic tissue could be found in the non-classic form of CAH with only mild androgen excess, we can only hypothesize that the true incidence of prostatic tissue in the female genital tract is likely underestimated. Therefore, the possibility of prostate tissue should always be considered as a differential diagnosis for atypical tissue in the female genital tract, especially in women with a history of some form of androgen excess. In this context, it would be interesting to determine whether ectopic prostatic tissue can also be found in patients with polycystic ovary syndrome. In addition, these case reports emphasize the need for adapted screening in female patients with any form of hyperandrogenemia, as malignant neoplasms of prostate tissue in these patients are possible.

Author Contributions: L.T., M.K.A., I.D., C.L., H.N., H.S. and N.R. provided data. N.G. performed the processing of the tissue samples and prepared the tissue images. L.T. and N.R. drafted the manuscript. All authors have read and agreed to the published version of the manuscript.

Funding: This work was supported by the Deutsche Forschungsgemeinschaft (DFG, German Research Foundation) project no. 314061271-TRR 205 and Heisenberg Professorship 325768017 to N.R., the German Ministry of Health (DSDCare 2519FSB503) to N.R., the International Fund raising Congenital Adrenal Hyperplasia/European Society for Pediatric Endocrinology project 2019 to N.R. and the Eva Luise und Horst Köhler Stiftung & Else Kröner-Fresenius-Stiftung 2019_KollegSE.03 to H N.

Institutional Review Board Statement: This work was conducted in accordance with the Declaration of Helsinki, and the protocol was approved by the Ethics Committee of the Medical Faculty of Ludwig Maximilians University Munich (Project number 19-558).

Informed Consent Statement: The written informed consent to publish images or other personal or clinical details of the patient was obtained from the patient. A copy of the consent form is available for review.

Data Availability Statement: The data of this case are available from the corresponding author upon reasonable request.

Acknowledgments: We thank the patient for consenting to this publication and Fatemeh Promoli for excellent technical support. This case report was prepared according to the CARE guidelines.

Conflicts of Interest: The authors declare no conflict of interest.

Abbreviations

17-OHP: 17-hydroxyprogesterone; 21-OHD: 21-hydroxylase deficiency; A4: androstenedione; ACTH: adrenocorticotropic hormone; CAH: congenital adrenal hyperplasia; DHEA-S: dehydroepiandrosterone sulfate; DSD: disorders of sexual development; E2: estradiol; FAI: free androgen index; FSH: follicle-stimulating hormone; HDE: hydrocortisone dose equivalent; HE: hematoxylin and eosin; HPV: human papillomavirus; LH: luteinizing hormone; P: measurement of pregnanetriol in 24-h urine sample; PSA: prostate specific antigen; SHBG: sex hormone binding globulin; T: testosterone.

References

1. Anderson, W.J.; Kolin, D.L.; Neville, G.; Diamond, D.A.; Crum, C.P.; Hirsch, M.S.; Vargas, S.O. Prostatic Metaplasia of the Vagina and Uterine Cervix: An Androgen-associated Glandular Lesion of Surface Squamous Epithelium. *Am. J. Surg. Pathol.* **2020**, *44*, 1040–1049. [CrossRef] [PubMed]
2. McCluggage, W.G.; Ganesan, R.; Hirschowitz, L.; Miller, K.; Rollason, T.P. Ectopic prostatic tissue in the uterine cervix and vagina: Report of a series with a detailed immunohistochemical analysis. *Am. J. Surg. Pathol.* **2006**, *30*, 209–215. [CrossRef] [PubMed]
3. Wesselius, R.; Schotman, M.; Schotman, M.; Pereira, A.M. A Patient (46XX) With Congenital Adrenal Hyperplasia and Prostate Cancer: A Case Report. *J. Endocr. Soc.* **2017**, *1*, 1213–1216. [CrossRef] [PubMed]
4. Elfekih, H.; Ben Abdelkrim, A.; Marzouk, H.; Saad, G.; Gasmi, A.; Gribaa, M.; Zaghouani, H.; Hasni, Y.; Maaroufi, A. Prostatic tissue in 46XX congenital adrenal hyperplasia: Case report and literature review. *Clin. Case Rep.* **2021**, *9*, 1655–1662. [CrossRef]
5. Fang, B.; Cho, F.; Lam, W. Prostate gland development and adrenal tumor in a female with congenital adrenal hyperplasia: A case report and review from radiology perspective. *J. Radiol. Case Rep.* **2013**, *7*, 21–34. [CrossRef]
6. Finkielstain, G.P.; Vieites, A.; Bergadá, I.; Rey, R.A. Disorders of Sex Development of Adrenal Origin. *Front. Endocrinol. (Lausann)* **2021**, *12*, 770782. [CrossRef]
7. Merke, D.P.; Auchus, R.J. Congenital Adrenal Hyperplasia Due to 21-Hydroxylase Deficiency. *N. Engl. J. Med.* **2020**, *383*, 1248–1261. [CrossRef]
8. Speiser, P.W.; Arlt, W.; Auchus, R.J.; Baskin, L.S.; Conway, G.S.; Merke, D.P.; Meyer-Bahlburg, H.F.L.; Miller, W.L.; Montori, V.M.; Oberfield, S.E.; et al. Congenital Adrenal Hyperplasia Due to Steroid 21-Hydroxylase Deficiency: An Endocrine Society Clinical Practice Guideline. *J. Clin. Endocrinol. Metab.* **2018**, *103*, 4043–4088. [CrossRef]
9. Wedell, A. Molecular genetics of 21-hydroxylase deficiency. *Endocr. Dev.* **2011**, *20*, 80–87.
10. Hannah-Shmouni, F.; Morissette, R.; Sinaii, N.; Elman, M.; Prezant, T.R.; Chen, W.; Pulver, A.; Merke, D.P. Revisiting the prevalence of nonclassic congenital adrenal hyperplasia in US Ashkenazi Jews and Caucasians. *Genet. Med. Off. J. Am. Coll. Med. Genet.* **2017**, *19*, 1276–1279. [CrossRef]
11. Nordenström, A.; Falhammar, H. Management of endocrine disease: Diagnosis and management of the patient with non-classic CAH due to 21-hydroxylase deficiency. *Eur. J. Endocrinol.* **2019**, *180*, R127–R145. [CrossRef] [PubMed]
12. New, M.I.; Abraham, M.; Gonzalez, B.; Dumic, M.; Razzaghy-Azar, M.; Chitayat, D.; Sun, L.; Zaidi, M.; Wilson, R.C.; Yuen, T. Genotype-phenotype correlation in 1507 families with congenital adrenal hyperplasia owing to 21-hydroxylase deficiency. *Proc. Natl. Acad. Sci. USA* **2013**, *110*, 2611–2616. [CrossRef] [PubMed]
13. Kiviat, M.D.; Leonard, J.M. True prostatic tissue in 46,XX female with adrenogenital syndrome. *Urology* **1978**, *12*, 75–78. [CrossRef]
14. Subramanian, S.; Gamanagatti, S.; Sharma, R.M.R. demonstration of a prostate gland in a female pseudohermaphrodite. *Pediatr. Radiol.* **2006**, *36*, 1194–1196. [CrossRef]
15. Lázaro, A.P.; de Lacerda, A.M.; Ghiaroni, J.; de Miranda, L.C.; Vidal, A.P.; Collett-Solberg, P.F.; Michelatto, D.P.; Mello, M.P.; Guimarães, M.M. Leydig cell tumour in a 46,XX child with congenital adrenal hyperplasia due to 21-hydroxylase deficiency. *Horm. Res. Paediatr.* **2013**, *79*, 179–184. [CrossRef]
16. Nucci, M.R.; Ferry, J.A.; Young, R.H. Ectopic prostatic tissue in the uterine cervix: A report of four cases and review of ectopic prostatic tissue. *Am. J. Surg. Pathol.* **2000**, *24*, 1224–1230. [CrossRef]
17. Winters, J.L.; Chapman, P.H.; Powell, D.E.; Banks, E.R.; Allen, W.R.; Wood, D.P., Jr. Female pseudohermaphroditism due to congenital adrenal hyperplasia complicated by adenocarcinoma of the prostate and clear cell carcinoma of the endometrium. *Am. J. Clin. Pathol.* **1996**, *106*, 660–664. [CrossRef]
18. Boutin, E.L.; Battle, E.; Cunha, G.R. The response of female urogenital tract epithelia to mesenchymal inductors is restricted by the germ layer origin of the epithelium: Prostatic inductions. *Differentiation* **1991**, *48*, 99–105. [CrossRef]
19. Singh, K.; Sung, C.J.; Lawrence, W.D.; Quddus, M.R. Testosterone-induced "Virilisation" of Mesonephric Duct Remnants and Cervical Squamous Epithelium in Female-to-Male Transgenders: A Report of 3 Cases. *Int. J. Gynecol. Pathol.* **2017**, *36*, 328–333. [CrossRef]
20. Paulino Mda, C.; Steinmetz, L.; Menezes Filho, H.C.; Kuperman, H.; Della Manna, T.; Vieira, J.G.; Blasbalg, R.; Baroni, R.; Setian, N.; Damiani, D. [Search of prostatic tissue in 46, XX congenital adrenal hyperplasia]. *Arq. Bras. Endocrinol. Metabol.* **2009**, *53*, 716–720.

21. Yeşilkaya, E.; Cinaz, P.; Bideci, A.; Camurdan, O.; Boyraz, M.A. 46XX disorder of sex development with a prostate gland and increased level of prostate-specific antigen. *J. Natl. Med. Assoc.* **2008**, *100*, 256–258. [CrossRef]
22. Delle Piane, L.; Rinaudo, P.F.; Miller, W.L. 150 years of congenital adrenal hyperplasia: Translation and commentary of De Crecchio's classic paper from 1865. *Endocrinology* **2015**, *156*, 1210–1217. [CrossRef] [PubMed]
23. Heyns, C.F.; Rimington, P.D.; Kurger, T.F.; Falck, V.G. Benign prostatic hyperplasia and uterine leiomyomas in a female pseudohermaphrodite: A case report. *J. Urol.* **1987**, *137*, 1245–1247. [CrossRef]
24. Klessen, C.; Asbach, P.; Hein, P.A.; Beyersdorff, D.; Hamm, B.; Taupitz, M. Complex genital malformation in a female with congenital adrenal hyperplasia: Evaluation with magnetic resonance imaging. *Acta Radiol.* **2005**, *46*, 891–894. [CrossRef]
25. Kim, K.R.; Park, K.H.; Kim, J.W.; Cho, K.J.; Ro, J.Y. Transitional cell metaplasia and ectopic prostatic tissue in the uterine cervix and vagina in a patient with adrenogenital syndrome: Report of a case suggesting a possible role of androgen in the histogenesis. *Int. J. Gynecol. Pathol.* **2004**, *23*, 182–187. [CrossRef]

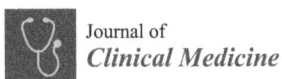

Journal of Clinical Medicine

Article

Identifying the Resource Needs of Young People with Differences of Sex Development

Gina Tonkin-Hill [1,2,*], Chloe Hanna [1,2,3], Roberto Bonelli [4], Rowena Mortimer [1,2], Michele A. O'Connell [1,2,3] and Sonia R. Grover [1,2,3,*]

[1] Faculty of Medicine, Dentistry and Health Sciences, University of Melbourne, Melbourne, VIC 3010, Australia; chloe.hanna@rch.org.au (C.H.); rowena.mortimer@gmail.com (R.M.); michele.o'connell@rch.org.au (M.A.O.)
[2] Department of Gynaecology, Royal Children's Hospital, Melbourne, VIC 3052, Australia
[3] Murdoch Children's Research Institute, Melbourne, VIC 3052, Australia
[4] Walter and Eliza Hall Institute, Melbourne, VIC 3052, Australia; bonelli.r@wehi.edu.au
* Correspondence: ginatonkinhill@gmail.com (G.T.-H.); sonia.grover@rch.org.au (S.R.G.)

Abstract: Adolescents with differences of sex development (DSD) often have complex medical, surgical, and psychological care needs and require age-appropriate resources. This cross-sectional study describes the past and current experiences of adolescents and young adults with DSD and their need for information and support. Participants aged 14–30 years with DSD diagnoses were identified, either from departmental records at the Royal Children's Hospital (RCH), Melbourne, Australia, or from the private practice of a gynaecologist linked to RCH. Anonymized data were collected from a specifically designed online survey. Of the 314 successfully traced patients, 91 (28.9%) completed the survey. Amongst respondents, older age was strongly correlated with higher levels of distress at the time of disclosure (b = 0.67, $p < 0.001$). People who reported greater understanding of their condition (b = −0.45, $p = 0.010$) and higher levels of support (b = −0.40, $p = 0.003$) identified lower levels of current distress. Respondents preferred to receive information from a specialist doctor, GP, or websites and reported information needs being highest during adolescence. Only one in four respondents recalled ever being offered psychological support. A number of perceived barriers to accessing support were identified. Our findings indicate that young people's information and support needs may be best met by improving online resources, as well as increasing introductions to knowledgeable and appropriate primary care physicians, psychological services, and peer support groups. Further work to promote and increase engagement with psychological and peer support for those with DSD will be important.

Keywords: differences of sex development; intersex; adolescent; young adult; disclosure; patient satisfaction; social support; psychological support systems

Citation: Tonkin-Hill, G.; Hanna, C.; Bonelli, R.; Mortimer, R.; O'Connell, M.A.; Grover, S.R. Identifying the Resource Needs of Young People with Differences of Sex Development. J. Clin. Med. 2022, 11, 4372. https://doi.org/10.3390/jcm11154372

Academic Editor: K. Katharina Rall

Received: 28 May 2022
Accepted: 22 July 2022
Published: 27 July 2022

Publisher's Note: MDPI stays neutral with regard to jurisdictional claims in published maps and institutional affiliations.

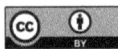

Copyright: © 2022 by the authors. Licensee MDPI, Basel, Switzerland. This article is an open access article distributed under the terms and conditions of the Creative Commons Attribution (CC BY) license (https://creativecommons.org/licenses/by/4.0/).

1. Introduction

Differences of sex development (DSD), alternatively known as disorders of sex development or intersex variations, are a group of congenital conditions in which developmental, chromosomal, gonadal, or anatomical sex is atypical [1]. Their phenotypical overlap adds to diagnostic complexity, which can lead to a delayed diagnosis or difficulty establishing a diagnosis [2,3]. Combined with their clinical diversity, this can result in inconsistent recommendations from different specialists and fragmentation of care [4]. Historically, as diagnoses are often made in childhood, decisions regarding treatment and care, including surgery for their congenital anomalies/variations, were made before the young person could participate and give informed consent. In the past, lack of understanding and social stigma has resulted in non-disclosure of diagnosis and further negative psychosocial effects [5].

Consensus statements support multidisciplinary teams (MDTs), open communication, and full disclosure [1,6,7]. Nevertheless, adolescents and young adults with DSD face complex issues. They need relevant age-appropriate information and support to adjust and cope with their diagnosis and its potential implications [7]. Puberty, with its increased risk for mental health problems, is when adolescents with DSD may become aware of their differences [8]. Some people require pubertal induction, which, in itself, may impact on psychological well-being [7,8], while others may learn of anatomical differences that will impact fertility. This increases their information and support needs at this time.

Previous studies indicate parental care, peer relations, experiencing social acknowledgement, feelings of normality and control, and access to specialist and psychological care contribute positively to psychological well-being [4,9,10]. General practitioners (GPs) are key to care coordination, and ideally, continuous liaison should occur between GPs and the MDT. Psychological and peer support have been shown to help young people develop coping strategies, promoting positive adaptation and assisting decisions about gender, surgery, and hormone replacement [1,10]. Previous research suggests that psychological support needs to be offered repeatedly, over time [11].

At the Royal Children's Hospital, Melbourne, Australia (RCH), children and adolescents with DSD are managed by a MDT comprising pediatric endocrinologists and surgeons (gynecology and urology), clinical geneticists, clinical ethicists, and a DSD clinical coordinator. The DSD coordinator provides primary liaison between the family and the MDT [12] and connects to online information, support groups, and psychologists in the community.

Self-reports from children and young adults about their information and support needs are required to guide optimal care planning. It is known that parents overestimate physical health while underestimating emotional health [13]. Due to the relative rarity of DSD conditions, studies to date have been limited by small sample sizes, and comparisons between different diagnoses are limited [10,14]. This study offers an insight into young people's resource needs with a moderate sample size including three sufficiently large diagnostic groups to be compared. We aimed to examine (i) the lived experience of participants relating to disclosure of their DSD, their levels of distress, and their understanding of their variation; (ii) participants' experience within the medical system; and (iii) participants' age-specific preferences for information and support, including primary physician care, psychological, and peer support.

2. Materials and Methods

The past and current experiences of adolescents and young adults with DSD were studied between February and May 2017. The cross-sectional study included young people aged 14–30 years with DSD diagnoses, as defined in the 2006 consensus statement [1], but it excluded those with significant intellectual disability or need for an interpreter. Potential participants were identified from the electronic medical record and departmental clinical lists and recruited by a researcher with no prior contact. The age and gender/sex of non-participants were collected from their file. Giving an email address and clicking on an emailed survey link implied consent [15]. Participants under 18 years required additional parent/guardian consent. RCH Human Research Ethics Committee (HREC37003) approved the research.

Patients were surveyed by using a specifically designed questionnaire delivered online [15]. Anonymized data were analyzed by using Excel 14.0.0 and R statistical software version 3.4.0. Inference on Likert scales was performed by using linear regression models employing a Wald test. The three largest diagnostic groups were used for comparisons: MRKH (Mayer–Rokitansky–Küster–Hauser), CAH (congenital adrenal hyperplasia), and TS (Turner syndrome). Differences in rate of participation were examined by using a binomial test for diagnoses and a chi-squared test for gender/sex and age. Distress was assessed by responding "strongly agree" or "agree" to feeling worried/troubled/distressed on a 5-point Likert scale. All linear regression models were corrected for potential confounding effects, and their results are presented in terms of regression coefficient (b) and p-value (p). The p-values < 0.05 are considered significant.

3. Results

3.1. Demographics

Of 438 potential participants, 314 were successfully contacted. Survey links were emailed to 116 people; 91 participants completed the survey.

Table 1 displays the diagnoses, age brackets, and gender for traced participants. The participation rate for people with MRKH (47.9%) was significantly higher than the general response rate (28.9%, $p = 0.006$). Males participated at a significantly lower rate (12.6%) than females (33.3%, $p < 0.001$). The numbers of people identifying with non-binary identities were too low to compare in this group. People <18 years participated at a significantly higher rate (47.4%) than people >18 years (10.2%, $p < 0.001$).

Table 1. Diagnosis, age (current and at diagnosis), and gender of survey participants; 0–4 years includes "as long as I can remember". DR = "I don't remember".

$n = 91$	Total	Current Age	Age at Learning of Diagnosis
		Years (Mean (SD))	Years (Mean (SD))
Age			
<18	16		
≥18	75		
Gender			
Female	78		
Male	11		
Intersex	2		
Diagnosis			
Congenital adrenal hyperplasia	17	21.4 (4.5)	3.5 (3.3)
Turner syndrome	18	21.7 (3.9)	6.7 (4.7)
MRKH	23	23.7 (3.2)	15.5 (2.3)
Androgen insensitivity	4	22.0 (6.1)	10.3 (6.2)
Bladder exstrophy	6	22.0 (5.8)	4.5 (3.8)
Cloacal anomalies	2	19.5 (2.5)	2 (0)
Gonadal dysgenesis	7	23.4 (4.4)	7.7 (6.8)
Primary ovarian insufficiency	7	25.6 (2.3)	16.3 (1.7)
Klinefelter syndrome	2	22.0 (0)	4.5 (2.5)
5-alpha reductase deficiency	1	17	17
Hypogonadotropic hypogonadism	1	17	12
Anorchia	2	17.0 (0)	7 (5)
VACTERL without uterus	1	27	2

The mean (SD) age of participants at completion of survey was 22.5(4.8) years. For the majority of their care, 58 participants reported care provided at our tertiary pediatric center, 21 in private consultations, 11 in another tertiary Australian hospital, and 1 overseas. All participants >18 years had completed high school. Two participants identified as Aboriginal. Currently, 78 respondents identify as female, 11 as male, and 2 as intersex. No participant reported previous gender incongruity; however, one "did not know" and nine did not respond. Sex was recalled as uncertain at birth in seven (8%) people, while six (7%) did not know. Of respondents, 80 were assigned female at birth, and 11 were male. Reassignment of sex occurred in two children (one male and one female), both aged <4 years.

3.2. Disclosure, Distress, and Understanding

Of participants, 41% were told about their DSD aged 0–4 years, 9% between 5 and 9 years, 18% between 10 and 14 years, and 31% between 15 and 19 years, while 2% did not remember. Of the 24 who were told aged 15–19 years, 6 had primary ovarian insufficiency (POI) and 16 had MRKH. The number of years (presented here as mean (SD)) since learning of their diagnosis for the largest diagnostic groups was 18.1 (5.7), 16.2 (7.3), and 9.0 (6.1) years for CAH, TS, and MRKH, respectively. Participants were first told about their DSD by their doctor (51%), their parent/guardian (34%), or other (15%).

The percentage and number of participants answering "strongly agree" or "agree" on a 5-point Likert scale to questions about distress, understanding and support is shown in Table 2. For the purposes of this study, "disclosure" refers to the time the participant learned of their DSD. Older age at the time of diagnosis correlated with greater initial distress (b = 0.67, $p < 0.001$). Adjusting for age, individuals with MRKH had significantly higher distress at disclosure compared to those with CAH (b = −2.0, $p < 0.001$) and TS (b = −2.1, $p < 0.001$). At disclosure, distress was not correlated with self-reported understanding of diagnosis (b = 0.10, $p = 0.43$).

Table 2. Percentage and number of participants answering "strongly agree" or "agree" on a 5-point Likert scale to questions on distress, understanding and support.

	%	N
At disclosure . . .		
I was given enough information	62%	44
I understood my DSD	49%	40
I felt worried/troubled/distressed	48%	38
Currently . . .		
I understand my DSD	82%	75
I feel worried/troubled/distressed	24%	22
I feel comfortable discussing my DSD with others	49%	43
I feel well supported	66%	58

Current distress correlated with higher distress at disclosure (b = 0.47, $p < 0.001$), lower self-reported understanding of their DSD (b = −0.45, $p = 0.010$), and not feeling supported (b = −0.40, $p = 0.003$). Current distress did not correlate with diagnosis or current age (b = 0.02, $p = 0.53$).

After adjusting for age, the group of participants with Turner syndrome had significantly higher current self-reported understanding of their diagnosis than those with CAH (b = −0.56, $p = 0.03$) and MRKH (−0.56, $p = 0.02$). Greater understanding of DSD correlated positively with feeling comfortable discussing their DSD with others (b = 0.46, $p = 0.02$).

3.3. Information and Support Needs

Of 86 respondents, the majority preferred to access information from their specialist doctor (81%), websites (51%), and general practitioner (48%). Respondents (n = 64) would have liked more information on a database of knowledgeable doctors (48%), tips on explaining to a new health professional (45%) or to others (39%), links to psychological support (45%) or peer support (34%), variety of treatment options (39%), fertility (36%), body diversity (30%), sexuality/intimate relationships (27%), sex education (22%), gender identity (20%), menstruation/periods (17%), and bladder and bowel function (13%). Desire for additional information correlated with current distress (b = 0.13, $p = 0.05$).

Health professionals that the respondents would have liked to have seen but have not seen in the past or currently are shown in Figure 1. The majority nominated counsellor and psychologist.

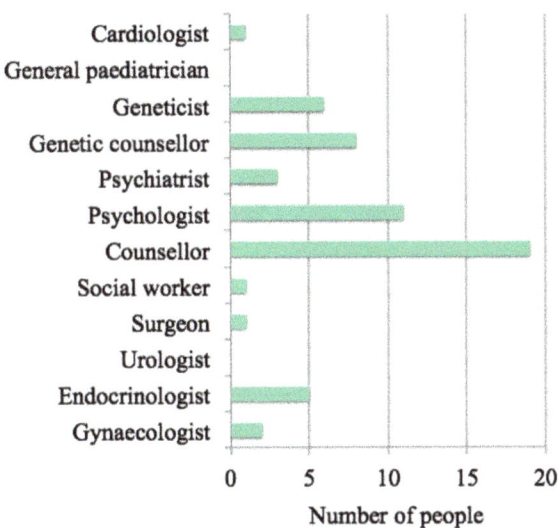

Figure 1. Health professionals that people would "at any stage have liked to have seen" but have not seen in the past or currently ($X^2 = 61.6, p < 0.0001$).

The age at which respondents would have preferred more information and access to health professionals is shown in Figure 2. For both, the peak request occurs between 15 and 19 years of age.

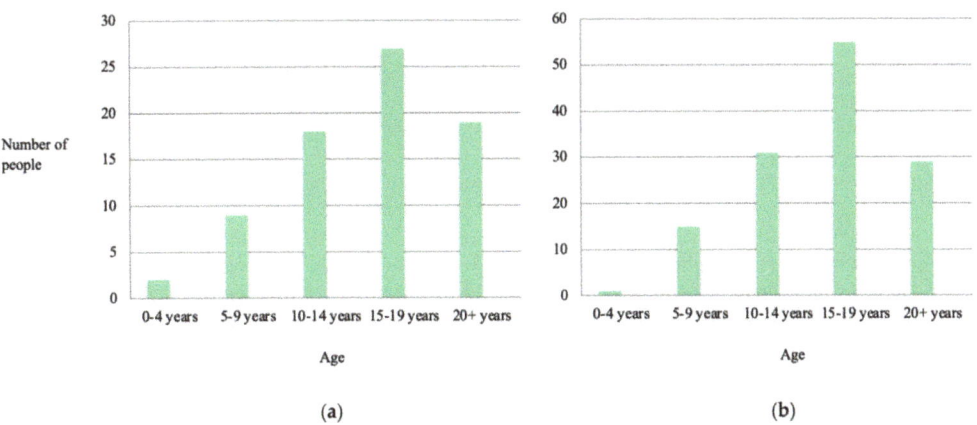

Figure 2. (a) Age at which participants would have liked to see any additional health professionals ($X^2 = 26.1, p < 0.0001$). (b) Age at which participants would have liked to access additional information ($X^2 = 59.4, p < 0.0001$).

Of 90 respondents, 63% discuss their DSD with a regular GP. Of those who do not ($n = 33$), 24% indicated they would like to. Related to their DSD, 49% have seen more than one GP, while 14% have never spoken to a GP. Of the 192 GPs seen by survey participants, 42% were considered helpful, 28% were considered unhelpful or lacking DSD information, and 31% were neutral or did not know. There was no correlation between distress and regular GP care ($b = -0.26, p = 0.36$). However, current distress significantly correlated with lower reported GP understanding ($b = -0.37, p = 0.02$).

Respondents (*n* = 84) felt supported by family (80%), specialist doctor (60%), friends (39%), partner (39%), GP (36%), psychologist (9%), or peer support group (7%). A minority of respondents (<5%) reported being supported by a psychiatrist, genetic counsellor, social worker, or social media. Feeling supported strongly correlated with participants feeling comfortable discussing their DSD with others (b = 0.61, $p < 0.001$).

Twenty-three (26%) participants recall being offered counselling or psychological support regarding their DSD. Participants who were offered psychological support, or who accessed it themselves, had significantly higher levels of distress at diagnosis (b = −2.64, $p = 0.01$). Of those who recall being offered psychological support, 83% did not use the service. The reasons included the following: they thought it would not help (68%), feeling they did not need it (11%), already accessing psychological care elsewhere (11%), embarrassment (5%), expense (5%), and long waiting times (5%). Of 83 respondents, 18% reported that their DSD affects their mental health, which correlated with their current DSD-related distress (b = 1.27, $p < 0.001$).

Of 18 (20%) respondents who had tried accessing peer support, 61% felt they were provided relevant information. Of these, 91% "strongly agree" or "agree" to peer support groups being helpful. Difficulty accessing peer support was reported by 50% (*n* = 9) of respondents. Respondents would prefer someone from the hospital introduced them (72%), to make contact themselves (11%), and did not know (17%). Respondents accessing peer support were significantly more distressed at diagnosis (b = 0.88, $p = 0.02$); however, this correlation disappeared when compared to current distress. Of 72 respondents (80%) who have not accessed peer support, 40% state that they did not need extra support, 38% preferred to deal with things on their own, 26% had never heard of peer support, 17% did not think it would help, 13% felt embarrassed, 1.4% were worried it was not confidential, and 10% did not know.

4. Discussion

This study affords important insights into the self-reported experiences and resource needs of a cohort of young people with DSD. While the majority reported high levels of support, significant opportunities for improvement are identified. Features associated with current distress included distress at disclosure, low understanding of their DSD, poor support, and lower GP understanding. Importantly for service provision, late adolescence was reported as the peak time when additional information, resources, and access to a broader range of clinicians is needed. With increasing independence, finishing school, and transitioning to adult services, this is known to be a time of change for young people [5].

This study supports the widespread recommendation for open communication and early disclosure of DSD diagnosis to enhance adaptive coping skills [1,7,16,17]. Older age at the time of disclosure correlated strongly with higher distress at disclosure. Distress may relate to the nature and implications of the diagnosis, as well as greater age-appropriate level of understanding. Higher distress at disclosure also correlates strongly with higher current distress, suggesting that earlier, more positive disclosure may prime for less distress in the future. However, for those with MRKH or POI, diagnosis is typically not apparent until adolescence, and, thus, the older age of disclosure is unavoidable.

The study found that, regardless of age at disclosure, those with a diagnosis of MRKH were more distressed than those with CAH or TS. Contributing factors may be that participants with CAH and TS learned of their diagnosis at a younger age and had longer to understand its impacts on their bodies and well-being. For people with MRKH, there is evidence that distress reduces with time from diagnosis [18], which may mirror the trajectory for those with CAH and TS reported here.

Compared to when they were diagnosed, participants' level of distress was improved, as was their understanding of their diagnosis. Current distress did not correlate with specific DSD or age. Interestingly, while distress did not correlate with level of understanding at disclosure, current distress correlated with current DSD understanding and level of support. This highlights that, while initial distress is influenced by the type of diagnosis and age, information and support needs gain importance over time.

Some participants, across a range of conditions, did not know whether their sex at birth was uncertain. The reported rate of uncertain sex at birth (8%) was also quite low, considering the high proportion of participants with CAH. We could infer that, although participants were likely given clear information about their health history, the uncertainty of sex at birth was not emphasized. These participants did not express increased distress regarding non-disclosure.

Significant developmental changes occur during adolescence [19]. People with DSD may experience extra social and emotional challenges associated with atypical anatomy, infertility, hormonal function, and genes [20]. In our cohort, participants preferred to access DSD information from their specialist doctor, GP, and websites. The desire for more information correlates with feeling distressed. This is a cross-sectional study, so it limits our ability to imply causality. Nonetheless, our results suggest that, with improved understanding, participants may feel less distressed, more comfortable speaking with others about their DSD, and also more supported.

The importance of support from a well-informed and regular GP is identified, although participants report difficulty accessing knowledgeable GPs. Similarly, the American Academy of Pediatrics [21] states that the absence of primary care involvement leads to expensive, episodic, and fragmented care. Young people can find explaining their condition to health professionals uncomfortable or burdensome, while GPs may have infrequent experience with DSDs and have difficulty finding sufficient information. Given the associations of lower distress with feeling well informed and supported, our data support efforts to improve information and resources for GPs. As young people also endorsed the use of trusted websites for information, online resources that they can share with their GP could also be helpful.

Stigmatization predisposes individuals to poor mental health [22]. Less than half of study participants felt comfortable discussing their DSD with others, and one-third felt unsupported. While participants reported that their main sources of support were family, specialist doctors, and GPs, they reported lower rates of support from friends and partners. It is not known if participants shared their diagnosis with friends and partners or whether they do not require their support. While current care models and advocacy groups seek to portray DSDs as part of the natural spectrum of development [23,24], there remains a general lack of awareness of DSD in society [25]. Almost half of participants would like to be linked to psychological support, and one-third would like information on peer support; these findings are similar to those of other studies [4,9,10].

While other studies have reported high rates of psychological distress [10,20], less than 20% of participants in this study reported their DSD affecting their mental health. This rate remains slightly higher than the global adolescent population [26]; however, this result concurs with previous research at RCH which found the physical and mental health of the DSD group to be similar to that of Hirschsprung and diabetes mellitus comparison groups [27]. Due to the self-selecting participation in these studies, those who were struggling may have been less likely to participate. Our study still indicates an unmet need for psychological support and perceived barriers to access. While a distressed minority recalled being offered psychological support, the majority did not. As our MDT does not include a psychologist (due to resource constraints); this may reflect genuinely low rates of referral and/or recall bias. Where offered, low rates of uptake of psychological support could also reflect participants' fear of non-DSD-specialized care and the effort involved in explaining their condition, as community psychologists' expertise in DSD management is often limited [20]. At our center, a DSD care coordinator, who was introduced a few years ago, provides support and resources to all children and young people and their families. The effect of this may not yet be present in this study. Our findings also support previous research recommending repetitive offers of psychological support [11]. Lastly, referrals to professionals with specific expertise are necessary where a dedicated psychologist is not part of the MDT, and, moving forward, a database of DSD-knowledgeable psychological professionals would be beneficial.

While only 20% of respondents reported seeking peer support, it was reported as helpful. Many found it difficult to make contact with peer support and stated that they would like to be introduced by the hospital. The correlation between distress and accessing peer support disappeared over time, indicating that peer support may partly decrease distress associated with diagnosis. While over a third of participants who had not accessed peer support stated that they did not need extra support, more than a quarter had never heard of a peer support group. This suggests the availability and potential benefits of peer support groups could be better promoted by the treating team and online.

Our study has a number of strengths and limitations. Adolescents and young adults were specifically targeted to explore ways to improve care pathways. The sample size was modest but relatively large compared to other DSD studies [10,20,28]. MRKH was the only group with significantly higher participation, and they reported the most distress at diagnosis. While MRKH participants were older at the time of diagnosis and may have had better recall, selection bias may have impacted this finding. Similar to other studies [10,28], the participation rates of males and of older patients were significantly lower. The number of female participants may be explained by the gynecology department's DSD database, which includes private gynecology patients. Older patients may have been less inclined to participate due to a lower sense of connection to their affiliated treating physician or hospital [28]. No recruitment from organizations or support groups occurred.

5. Conclusions

Adolescents with differences of sex development often have complex medical and psychological care needs and require age-appropriate resources. This study informs future care planning and areas for improvement related to the specific information and psychosocial support needs of adolescents with DSD and their preferences for connection with support services. Low access to and uptake of psychological support and an unmet desire for information in the teenage years was identified. Importantly, people who reported greater understanding of their condition and higher levels of support had lower levels of current distress. This key finding underscores the importance of ensuring young people are well informed in relation to their bodies and the potential implications of their DSD. Preferred methods of accessing information were from a specialist doctor, GP, or websites. Barriers still exist for people wanting to connect with psychosocial supports, even when this support is offered. Our findings outline the importance of providing regular opportunities for peer and professional psychosocial supports, as well as improving individual, GP, and other healthcare professional knowledge of DSD to optimally support this potentially vulnerable cohort.

Author Contributions: Conceptualization, S.R.G., M.A.O. and C.H.; methodology, R.B. and G.T.-H.; software, R.B.; validation, G.T.-H.; formal analysis, R.B. and G.T.-H.; investigation, G.T.-H. and R.M.; resources, S.R.G., M.A.O., C.H. and R.M.; data curation, G.T.-H.; writing—original draft preparation, G.T.-H.; writing—review and editing, G.T.-H., R.B., R.M., C.H., M.A.O. and S.R.G.; visualization, G.T.-H.; supervision, C.H., M.A.O. and S.R.G.; project administration, G.T.-H., R.M. and C.H.; funding acquisition, S.R.G. All authors have read and agreed to the published version of the manuscript.

Funding: This research received no external funding.

Institutional Review Board Statement: The study was conducted in accordance with the Declaration of Helsinki and approved by the Human Research Ethics Committee of the Royal Children's Hospital, Melbourne, Australia (HREC37003, 24/02/2017).

Informed Consent Statement: Informed consent was obtained from all subjects involved in the study.

Data Availability Statement: The data are not publicly available to maintain participant confidentiality.

Conflicts of Interest: The authors declare no conflict of interest.

References

1. Hughes, I.A.; Houk, C.; Ahmed, S.F.; Lee, P.A.; Society, L.W.P.E. Consensus statement on management of intersex disorders. *Arch. Dis. Child.* **2006**, *91*, 554–563. [CrossRef] [PubMed]
2. Ahmed, S.F.; Achermann, J.; Alderson, J.; Crouch, N.S.; Elford, S.; Hughes, I.A.; Krone, N.; McGowan, R.; Mushtaq, T.; O'Toole, S.; et al. Society for Endocrinology UK Guidance on the initial evaluation of a suspected difference or disorder of sex development (Revised 2021). *Clin. Endocrinol.* **2021**, *95*, 818–840. [CrossRef] [PubMed]
3. Barseghyan, H.; Délot, E.C.; Vilain, E. New technologies to uncover the molecular basis of disorders of sex development. *Mol. Cell Endocrinol.* **2018**, *468*, 60–69. [CrossRef] [PubMed]
4. Thyen, U.; Lux, A.; Jürgensen, M.; Hiort, O.; Köhler, B. Utilization of health care services and satisfaction with care in adults affected by disorders of sex development (DSD). *J. Gen. Intern. Med.* **2014**, *29* (Suppl. S3), S752–S759. [CrossRef]
5. Crouch, N.S.; Creighton, S.M. Transition of care for adolescents with disorders of sex development. *Nat. Rev. Endocrinol.* **2014**, *10*, 436–442. [CrossRef]
6. Lee, P.A.; Nordenström, A.; Houk, C.P.; Ahmed, S.F.; Auchus, R.; Baratz, A.; Dalke, K.B.; Liao, L.-M.; Lin-Su, K.; Looijenga, L.; et al. Global Disorders of Sex Development Update since 2006: Perceptions, Approach and Care. *Horm. Res. Paediatr.* **2016**, *85*, 158–180. [CrossRef]
7. Nordenström, A. Psychosocial Factors in Disorders of Sex Development in a Long-Term Perspective: What Clinical Opportunities are there to Intervene? *Horm. Metab. Res.* **2015**, *47*, 351–356. [CrossRef] [PubMed]
8. Kleinemeier, E.; Jürgensen, M.; Lux, A.; Widenka, P.-M.; Thyen, U. Psychological adjustment and sexual development of adolescents with disorders of sex development. *J. Adolesc. Health* **2010**, *47*, 463–471. [CrossRef] [PubMed]
9. Immelt, S. Psychological adjustment in young children with chronic medical conditions. *J. Pediatr. Nurs.* **2006**, *21*, 362–377. [CrossRef]
10. Schweizer, K.; Brunner, F.; Gedrose, B.; Handford, C.; Richter-Appelt, H. Coping With Diverse Sex Development: Treatment Experiences and Psychosocial Support During Childhood and Adolescence and Adult Well-Being. *J. Pediatr. Psychol.* **2016**, *42*, 504–519. [CrossRef]
11. Engberg, H.; Möller, A.; Hagenfeldt, K.; Nordenskjöld, A.; Frisén, L. The experience of women living with Congenital Adrenal Hyperplasia: Impact of the condition and the care given. *Clin. Endocrinol.* **2016**, *85*, 21–28. [CrossRef] [PubMed]
12. Royal Children's Hospital. Gynaecology. Available online: http://www.rch.org.au/rch_gynaecology/for_young_women/ (accessed on 28 September 2016).
13. Jürgensen, M.; Lux, A.; Wien, S.B.; Kleinemeier, E.; Hiort, O.; Thyen, U. Health-related quality of life in children with disorders of sex development (DSD). *Eur. J. Pediatr.* **2014**, *173*, 893–903. [CrossRef] [PubMed]
14. Amaral, R.C.; Inacio, M.; Brito, V.N.; Bachega, T.A.; Domenice, S.; Arnhold, I.J.; Madureira, G.; Gomes, L.; Costa, E.; Mendonca, B. Quality of life of patients with 46,XX and 46,XY disorders of sex development. *Clin. Endocrinol.* **2015**, *82*, 159–164. [CrossRef] [PubMed]
15. Resource Needs of Adolescents. Available online: https://redcap.mcri.edu.au/surveys/?s=JYNMKP4T93 (accessed on 27 April 2021).
16. Nordenström, A.; Thyen, U. Improving the communication of healthcare professionals with affected children and adolescents. *Endocr. Dev.* **2014**, *27*, 113–127. [PubMed]
17. American Academy of Pediatrics Committee on Pediatrics AIDS. Disclosure of illness status to children and adolescents with HIV infection. *Pediatrics* **1999**, *103*, 164–166.
18. Kimberley, N.; Hutson, J.M.; Southwell, B.R.; Grover, S.R. Well-being and sexual function outcomes in women with vaginal agenesis. *Fertil. Steril.* **2011**, *95*, 238–241. [CrossRef] [PubMed]
19. Suris, J.-C.; Michaud, P.-A.; Viner, R. The adolescent with a chronic condition. Part I: Developmental issues. *Arch. Dis. Child.* **2004**, *89*, 938–942. [CrossRef] [PubMed]
20. Liao, L.-M.; Tacconelli, E.; Wood, D.; Conway, G.; Creighton, S.M. Adolescent girls with disorders of sex development: A needs analysis of transitional care. *J. Pediatr. Urol.* **2010**, *6*, 609–613. [CrossRef] [PubMed]
21. American Academy of Pediatrics Council on Children with Disabilities. Care coordination in the medical home: Integrating health and related systems of care for children with special health care needs. *Pediatrics* **2005**, *116*, 1238–1244. [CrossRef]
22. Liao, L.-M.; Simmonds, M. A values-driven and evidence-based health care psychology for diverse sex development. *Psychol. Sex.* **2014**, *5*, 83–101. [CrossRef]
23. Cools, M.; Nordenström, A.; Robeva, R.; Hall, J.; Westerveld, P.; Flück, C.; Köhler, B.; Berra, M.; Springer, A.; Schweizer, K.; et al. Caring for individuals with a difference of sex development (DSD): A Consensus Statement. *Nat. Rev. Endocrinol.* **2018**, *14*, 415–429. [CrossRef] [PubMed]
24. Darlington Statement. 2017. Available online: https://darlington.org.au/statement/ (accessed on 26 May 2022).
25. Rolston, A.M.; Gardner, M.; Vilain, E.; Sandberg, D.E. Parental Reports of Stigma Associated with Child's Disorder of Sex Development. *Int. J. Endocrinol.* **2015**, *2015*, 980121. [CrossRef] [PubMed]
26. Adolescent Mental Health. Available online: https://www.who.int/news-room/fact-sheets/detail/adolescent-mental-health (accessed on 26 May 2022).

27. Warne, G.; Grover, S.; Hutson, J.; Sinclair, A.; Metcalfe, S.; Northam, E.; Freeman, J.; Murdoch Childrens Research Institut. A long-term outcome study of intersex conditions. *J. Pediatr. Endocrinol. Metab.* **2005**, *18*, 555–567. [CrossRef] [PubMed]
28. Lux, A.; Kropf, S.; Kleinemeier, E.; Jürgensen, M.; Thyen, U. Clinical evaluation study of the German network of disorders of sex development (DSD)/intersexuality: Study design, description of the study population, and data quality. *BMC Public Health* **2009**, *9*, 110. [CrossRef] [PubMed]

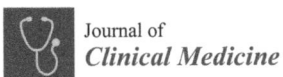

Review

An Interdisciplinary Approach to Müllerian Outflow Tract Obstruction Associated with Cloacal Malformation and Cloacal Exstrophy

Bryan S. Sack [1,*], K. Elizabeth Speck [2], Anastasia L. Hryhorczuk [3], David E. Sandberg [4], Kate H. Kraft [1], Matthew W. Ralls [2], Catherine E. Keegan [5], Elisabeth H. Quint [6] and Melina L. Dendrinos [6]

1. Department of Urology, Division of Pediatric Urology, University of Michigan, Ann Arbor, MI 48109, USA; kraftk@med.umich.edu
2. Department of Surgery, Section of Pediatric Surgery, University of Michigan, Ann Arbor, MI 48109, USA; speckk@med.umich.edu (K.E.S.); mralls@med.umich.edu (M.W.R)
3. Department of Radiology, University of Michigan, Ann Arbor, MI 48109, USA; ahryhorc@med.umich.edu
4. Department of Pediatrics, Division of Pediatric Psychology, University of Michigan, Ann Arbor, MI 48109, USA; dsandber@med.umich.edu
5. Department of Pediatrics, Division of Pediatric Genetics, Metabolism, and Genomic Medicine, University of Michigan, Ann Arbor, MI 48109, USA; keeganc@med.umich.edu
6. Department of Obstetrics and Gynecology, University of Michigan, Ann Arbor, MI 48109, USA; equint@med.umich.edu (E.H.Q.); mdendrin@med.umich.edu (M.L.D.)
* Correspondence: bsack@med.umich.edu; Tel.: +1-734-615-1260; Fax: +1-734-615-3520

Citation: Sack, B.S.; Speck, K.E.; Hryhorczuk, A.L.; Sandberg, D.E.; Kraft, K.H.; Ralls, M.W.; Keegan, C.E.; Quint, E.H.; Dendrinos, M.L. An Interdisciplinary Approach to Müllerian Outflow Tract Obstruction Associated with Cloacal Malformation and Cloacal Exstrophy. J. Clin. Med. 2022, 11, 4408. https://doi.org/10.3390/jcm11154408

Academic Editor: K. Katharina Rall

Received: 14 June 2022
Accepted: 21 July 2022
Published: 28 July 2022

Publisher's Note: MDPI stays neutral with regard to jurisdictional claims in published maps and institutional affiliations.

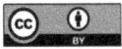

Copyright: © 2022 by the authors. Licensee MDPI, Basel, Switzerland. This article is an open access article distributed under the terms and conditions of the Creative Commons Attribution (CC BY) license (https://creativecommons.org/licenses/by/4.0/).

Abstract: People with cloacal malformation and 46,XX cloacal exstrophy are at risk of developing Müllerian outflow tract obstruction (OTO). Management of OTO requires expertise of many medical and surgical specialties. The primary presenting symptom associated with OTO is cyclical and later continuous pain and can be initially quelled with hormonal suppression as a temporizing measure to allow for patient maturation. The decision for timing and method of definitive treatment to establish a patent outflow tract that can also be used for penetrative sexual activity and potential fertility is a complicated one and incredibly variable based on patient age alone. To understand the management approach to OTO, we put forth five phases with associated recommendations: (1) caregiver and patient education and evaluation before obstruction; (2) presentation, diagnosis, and symptom temporization; (3) readiness assessment; (4) peri-procedural management; (5) long-term surveillance. This review will emphasize the importance of interdisciplinary team management of the complex shared medical, surgical, and psychological decision making required to successfully guide developing patients with outflow obstruction secondary to cloacal malformations and cloacal exstrophy through adolescence.

Keywords: cloacal malformation; cloacal exstrophy; vaginal obstruction; fertility; congenital anomalies; shared decision making

1. Introduction

Congenital anomalies of the reproductive tract resulting in Müllerian outflow tract obstruction (OTO) are rare and quite varied in terms of anatomy, presentation, and treatment [1], requiring the expertise of many medical and surgical specialties. OTO in patients without associated anomalies of the external genitalia usually presents unexpectedly during adolescence with cyclical or recurrent abdominopelvic pain and primary amenorrhea [2,3]. In individuals with associated early-diagnosed and reconstructed congenital anomalies, such as cloacal malformation and cloacal exstrophy, there is usually awareness by caregivers and healthcare providers of the potential for developing OTO in adolescence. Even with surgical creation of a potential outflow tract in early childhood for later menstrual flow, many of these patients will present with OTO in adolescence [4,5].

The primary presenting symptom associated with OTO is cyclical and later continuous pain and can be initially quelled with hormonal suppression as a temporizing measure to allow for patient maturation [6]. In addition, OTO may allow for neither penetrative sexual activity nor conception, whether spontaneous or assisted.

The decision for timing and method of definitive treatment to establish a patent outflow tract that can also be used for penetrative sexual activity and potential fertility is a complicated one and incredibly variable based on patient age and level of maturity. It requires thorough evaluation of anatomy, likelihood to have or desire future fertility, patient readiness for reconstruction and postoperative dilation if indicated, and, in some instances, gender identity. Family support is crucial to determine how and when to manage the OTO. Management discussions include long-term menstrual suppression, removal or reconstruction of uterine structure(s), and vaginoplasty. During initial evaluation, the healthcare team must be aware of the potential psychological, psychosocial, and psychosexual effects OTO may have had on the patient. This emphasizes the need for a biopsychosocial management strategy [7] rather than strictly a biomedical approach.

Interdisciplinary management is imperative to guide patients through the multifaceted process of treating the OTO. Each specialty within the interdisciplinary team works together jointly with the other disciplines while emphasizing their own specific skillset to create a coherent and encompassing strategy to the approach and management [8] (Table 1). This review will emphasize the importance of interdisciplinary team management of the complex shared medical, surgical, and psychological decision making required to successfully guide developing patients with outflow obstruction secondary to cloacal malformations and cloacal exstrophy through adolescence.

Table 1. Medical and Surgical Specialty Involvement at the Different Phases of Müllerian Outflow Tract Obstruction (specialties listed in alphabetical order).

Caregiver and Patient Education and Evaluation before Obstruction	Presentation, Diagnosis, and Symptom Temporization	Readiness Assessment	Peri-Procedural Management	Long-Term Surveillance
Gynecology	Endocrinology	Genetics	Gynecology	Gynecology
Pediatric Surgery	Gynecology	Gynecology	Pediatric Surgery	Maternal Fetal Medicine
Primary Care	Primary Care	Primary Care	Plastic Surgery	Previous Surgical Team
Psychology	Radiology	Psychology	Primary Care	Primary Care
Urology		Social Work	Psychology	Psychology
			Radiology	Reproductive Endocrinology and Infertility
			Social work	
			Urology	

2. Congenital Müllerian Anomalies at Risk for Outflow Obstruction

This review will focus on two congenital anomalies that are diagnosed early in life that have an increased risk of developing Müllerian outflow tract obstruction in adolescence.

Cloacal malformation has an incidence of 1 in 25,000 live female births. The perineal anatomy includes an imperforate anus with a single opening known as the common channel, which is a confluence of the rectum, vagina(s), and urinary system. These children require urgent fecal diversion with a colostomy and may require a vesicostomy or more often a vaginostomy [9] to allow for adequate urinary drainage, particularly if there is significant hydronephrosis or hydrocolpos. After these temporizing procedures, the infant will undergo separation of the rectal component with anorectoplasty using a posterior sagittal incision or an abdominal approach (open or laparoscopic), typically in the first year of life. Because of the high risk of future OTO after early reconstruction, the decision to perform a vaginoplasty at the time of the anorectoplasty has been questioned. With recent advancements of minimally invasive techniques, some have begun deferring vaginal reconstruction until adolescence because of this risk [10,11].

Vaginoplasty techniques at this age include total or partial urogenital mobilization (i.e., the urinary system and vagina are mobilized to the perineum with or without local skin flapping) or using a large or small bowel interposition to serve as a neovagina. Independent of the technique or decision to perform a vaginoplasty, appropriate delineation of the complete Müllerian tract anatomy is often fraught with difficulty. To highlight the frequency of more complicated anatomy, duplicated proximal vaginas are expected to be identified in 44–63% [5,12]. Furthermore, when surveyed, surgeons were uncertain of the Müllerian anatomy in 13–39% of cases after performing infant reconstruction [5,12]. This anatomical uncertainty, paired with less than desirable functional outcomes, emphasizes the need to rethink the timing of Müllerian reconstruction and highlights the need for longitudinal assessment of these patients for OTO as they enter adolescence.

Cloacal exstrophy has an incidence of 1 in nearly 200,000 male and female live births [13]. This anomaly consists of a midline anatomical defect that results in two separate exstrophied bladder plates laterally with a midline exstrophied cecal plate and often intussuscepted distal small bowel. This results in exposed and continuous urinary and fecal drainage. Like patients with cloacal malformation, these children require neonatal fecal diversion with an end colostomy, preserving any available colon. These patients also have an omphalocele, which is typically managed at the time of their fecal diversion. In late infancy, after these temporizing measures, the bladder and lower abdominal wall are closed to create a bladder. This anomaly is also referred to as OEIS complex (omphalocele-exstrophy-imperforate anus-spinal defects) because of the other concomitant anomalies.

Müllerian duct anatomy also varies widely in patients with 46,XX cloacal exstrophy. In one of the largest retrospective series of 30 patients, 43% (13/30) had vaginal and uterine duplication, and of the 47% (14/30) with a single vagina, five had vaginal atresia, and one had lateral displacement [14]. Like those with a cloacal malformation, many of these patients had uncertain anatomy after evaluation in the operating room [14]. For those with identifiable Müllerian anatomy, reconstruction is often pursued at the time of bladder reconstruction in late infancy. This may range from simply incising or removing a vaginal septum between two vaginas to intestinal interposition if the vagina is unable to reach the perineum. If the anatomy appears atretic or too complex for surgical reconstruction, hemi- and complete hysterectomies have been performed during early reconstruction [14–16]. However, there are many patients who did not undergo vaginal manipulation at the time of bladder closure, and all of these patients should be monitored closely into and through adolescence.

Although the gastrointestinal and urologic concerns are high priorities early in life, as these children age into adolescence, it is paramount that caregivers, patients, and the primary care providers appreciate the complex and uncertain vaginal and uterine anatomy that may later present with OTO.

3. Phases of Müllerian Outflow Tract Obstruction

To understand the different management aspects of outflow tract obstruction, we put forth *five phases* with included management recommendations (Table 2):

1. Caregiver and patient education and evaluation before obstruction;
2. Presentation, diagnosis, and symptom temporization;
3. Readiness assessment;
4. Peri-procedural management;
5. Long-term surveillance.

Table 2. Management Recommendations at the Different Phases of Müllerian Outflow Tract Obstruction.

Caregiver and Patient Education and Evaluation before Obstruction	Presentation, Diagnosis, and Symptom Temporization	Readiness Assessment	Peri-Procedural Management	Long-Term Surveillance
Shared decision making about potential OTO at initial reconstruction	Symptom assessment	Re-evaluation of pain management	Establish sexual activity goals	Evaluate recurrence of obstruction
Education about potential OTO at regular clinic visits	Ultrasound followed by MRI	Discuss desire and options for future fertility	Establish goals for fertility preservation	Determine need for continued vaginal dilation
Pelvic ultrasounds starting about 18 months after thelarche, every 6 months to evaluate for silent OTO	Pain control with hormonal suppression	Assess ability to perform vaginal dilation	Determine specific location of obstruction (may require additional imaging/endoscopy)	Perform regular PAP smears and contraception counseling
Evaluate past surgical details at thelarche to understand Müllerian anatomy	Evaluate past surgical details	Evaluate psychologic well-being and support system	Referral to genetics to discuss heritability	Assess sexuality and refer to psychology if concerns arise
			Create and move forward with an agreed upon surgical plan	Pre-conception counseling with REI, MFM, and surgical specialists
				Surgical assistance at time of cesarean delivery

OTO, outflow tract obstruction; MRI, magnetic resonance imaging; REI, reproductive endocrinology and infertility; MFM, maternal fetal medicine.

3.1. Caregiver and Patient Education and Evaluation before Obstruction

It is the responsibility of the care team to try and predict future OTO in children with cloacal exstrophy and cloacal malformation before they develop symptoms. This consideration and discussion should begin prior to initial infant reconstruction as part of the shared decision-making process that should include the future risk of OTO. Robust and repeated education should be provided at regular clinic visits for the caregivers and, beginning as early as mid-late childhood, with the patient about the possibility of developing OTO and the associated symptoms. During this pre-obstruction phase, assessment of patient maturity and addressing their emotional needs and potential reactions surrounding the understanding of their diagnosis will help with the readiness assessment at the time of OTO.

Around the time of breast development, even in the absence of OTO symptoms, the reconstructed anatomy should be reviewed to refamiliarize the team of the Müllerian anatomy at the time of initial surgical intervention. Ideally, the surgical team will remain involved in the long-term care given the anatomical variability of each patient. When this is not possible, the past surgical records should be reviewed in detail. It is recommended that about 18 months after thelarche (breast budding) or at least at breast Tanner stage 3, pelvic ultrasounds (US) are obtained every 6 months to evaluate for hematocolpos and/or hematometra, so menstrual suppression can be initiated if either are present [5]. Unfortunately, the OTO is usually diagnosed in a symptomatic state.

3.2. Presentation, Diagnosis, and Symptom Temporization

Presentation and diagnosis of OTO is established with clinical history, physical exam, imaging, and an understanding of previous surgical interventions, which is paramount to the eventual understanding of the extent of the outflow obstruction. The symptoms associated with outflow obstruction of menses may initially be nonspecific cyclical or non-cyclical abdominal pain, nausea, and generalized gastrointestinal or urinary symptoms and can easily be confused for appendicitis, ovarian torsion, constipation, passing of a kidney stone, or a urinary tract infection. Alternatively, patients may present with primary amenorrhea or dysmenorrhea with menses. Progressive cyclical pain should raise the suspicion of an outflow obstruction.

Upon presentation, a gentle external genital exam can be considered, dependent upon the patient's age and comfort level of the patient and their family. Child Life assistance should be considered. External inspection with mild labial retraction can identify the urethra, clitoris, presence of labia, a hymenal opening, and vaginal and rectal openings as well as their reconstructed anatomic relationship to each other. A digital rectal exam, if tolerated, can elucidate a low anterior bulge consistent with an outflow tract obstruction.

Adolescents with a suspected OTO should receive a transabdominal US as their initial imaging evaluation. US is a readily available and well-tolerated imaging modality that avoids both sedation and ionizing radiation. When an OTO is present, the US will demonstrate a distended vagina and/or uterus with low-level internal echoes compatible with blood products. The uterus or uteri can be identified superiorly with or without a cervical impression at the upper aspect of the vagina. Hematosalpinx, or blood-filled fallopian tubes, may also be appreciated, as the blood can pass retrograde. Often, the obstruction is large or complex, and US may not be able to delineate the obstruction clearly. If US findings are unclear or support OTO, a pelvic MRI is recommended shortly thereafter to further delineate the anatomy. An MRI provides excellent tissue characterization and allows for definitive characterization of blood products, which demonstrate hyperintense signal on T1-weighted sequences. It will also better define uterine and vaginal anatomy and their relationship with bowel neovagina if present. The radiological studies should be discussed with the radiologists and care team in detail. These imaging studies should confirm the outflow tract obstruction; however, additional imaging, exam under anesthesia, and endoscopic assessment may be required prior to any further planned interventions or suppression.

While the diagnosis is established, attempts to resolve the patient's pain using menstrual suppression should be made. Dependent on age and institutional referral patterns, this can be accomplished by the gynecology or pediatric endocrinology teams. Menstrual suppression can be achieved with continuous estrogen-progestin or progestin-only options. In refractory cases, GnRH agonists or antagonists can be considered, often initially in concert with other hormonal suppression or add-back therapy. Complete menstrual suppression is difficult to obtain, and the patient and family should be made aware. Even with successful suppression, the patient's pain often resolves slowly, and recurrence of pain requires diligent follow-up to identify the underlying cause. Continued pain can be secondary to additional menstrual break through bleeding in an obstructed space [6]; these patients will need re-evaluation. If pain remains an issue, often due to breakthrough bleeding, then continued retrograde menstruation can lead to further endometriosis and affect fertility. The care team should exhaust all possibilities for menstrual suppression, as this provides versatility in management strategies and the ability to delay definitive surgical management until the anatomy is well-defined and the patient feels ready, as determined by the readiness assessment.

3.3. Readiness Assessment

Once these adolescents have been diagnosed with an obstruction, and their symptoms have quiesced, the decision regarding if, how, and when to surgically intervene is not algorithmic. Prior to making this complex decision, there are factors that must be considered in this specific patient population. We use shared decision making among the patient, caregivers, and healthcare providers [17]. The primary factors that one must consider when performing the readiness assessment are pain management; desire, ability, and options for future fertility; ability to perform vaginal dilation before or after surgery; and psychological well-being and support system.

To navigate this readiness assessment, it is most beneficial when performed collaboratively in an interdisciplinary setting. We feel that the factors listed above make them the ideal candidates for the interdisciplinary nature of the DSD clinic, as it can address each of these concerns utilizing the expertise from the specific indicated specialists, which may include endocrinology, genetics, gynecology, plastic surgery, psychology, surgery, and urology.

Factors to Consider during Readiness Assessment

Pain Management—If the pain does not resolve with hormonal suppression, surgical correction may need to be undertaken more urgently prior to optimal patient readiness. Interventional radiology or surgical assistance with percutaneous vaginal or uterine drainage may help with symptom management; however, it is not definitive and has a possible infection risk [18]. Intervening too early with surgical reconstruction has been shown to have an increased failure rate secondary to inability to manage post-op vaginal dilation [10,19,20]. Although menstrual suppression allows for delay in intervention, there may be a longer time to resolution of pain compared to early surgery [6].

Desire, Ability, and Options for Future Fertility—Predicting the ability to conceive and carry a pregnancy to term with safe delivery in a person with a history of OTO is complicated. Many patients have already had multiple abdominal operations, leading to adhesions that may affect tubal patency. There are no cases in the current literature that describe successful pregnancy in a case of OTO with the presence of a bowel neovagina. Due to the hematometrocolpos that typically occurs, these patients experience significant retrograde menstruation into the pelvis and have higher frequency of endometriosis, which is another known risk factor for infertility [21,22]. Additionally, assessing cervical competency in these obstructed systems, even with MRI and endoscopy, is challenging. Based on the findings of limited retrospective outcome data from two case series in adult cloacal malformation patients without a history of OTO, 6 of 24 were able to have children (5 by cesarean delivery, 1 vaginally) [12], and 2 of 3 sexually active 46,XX cloacal exstrophy patients were able to conceive [14]. These details help counsel and direct the surgical decision to perform uterine-preserving interventions. Additional important pregnancy considerations include the higher likelihood of preterm labor and the recommendation for a cesarean delivery, which is considerably more complicated because of their variant anatomy and history of multiple pelvic surgeries [23]. The cesarean deliveries are often done with a surgical team approach.

Ability to Perform Vaginal Dilation—A major aspect that complicates the outcome and success of vaginal reconstruction is patient participation with vaginal dilation. Stenosis is common after vaginal reconstruction and long-term postoperative dilation is needed to prevent stenosis. The ability to self-dilate the vagina or neovagina requires an understanding of one's own anatomy, why the procedure was performed, and the necessity for long-term dilation. In early teens, this is physically, emotionally, and psychologically difficult and often results in non-compliance resulting in vaginal stenosis. Thorough counseling with the gynecology, surgery, urology, and psychology teams will hopefully preoperatively predict the inclination and ability to dilate, as many young adolescents are not emotionally ready to perform dilations, and some may not have adequate privacy [24]. Although the patient data are heterogenous in diagnosis, age, and surgical method, the success of vaginoplasty outcomes are improved when they are performed after puberty [10,19,20]. This is believed to stem from compliance with dilation and also estrogenization of the tissue during the post-operative healing process. Many recommend only undertaking these procedures when the patients are ready to initiate vaginal sexual activity [10,19,25]. We feel that the timing for intervention should be informed by the patient's interests for intimate vaginal activities with or without a partner. However, the prerequisite of being sexually active prior to offering vaginoplasty may be misguided because patients may be avoiding intimate interactions because of their atypical anatomy.

Psychologic Well-being and Support System—Determining readiness for a complex surgical reconstruction during the pubertal maturation period requires assessment of the patient's psychological well-being and the available support around the person. Fortunately, although those with complex anatomies such as cloacal exstrophy and cloacal malformation have other co-morbidities, they are reported to have good psychological functioning [26]. They are also able to socially integrate and adapt as adults [27]; however, adolescents may have anxiety about their genital appearance and sexual activity [27], which further emphasizes the need to inquire about their psychological, psychosocial, and psychosexual thoughts and concerns prior to moving forward with decision making. To help gain an understanding of this, we recommend that they undergo psychological evaluation prior to moving forward with surgical intervention. Utilization of social work support can help provide an understanding of the family and community network that can be used to help with decision making and post-operative care plans. Ensuring a stable support system in the early stages of surgical planning is critical and embarking on these types of interventions independently is discouraged.

At the end of the readiness assessment, the patient should be confident in moving forward with surgery to relieve the OTO. If the patient is not ready to move forward, reassessing periodically (e.g., every 6–12 months or based on symptomatology) is recommended.

These varying factors are intricately woven together and require the skills of many specialties to create a cohesive individualized management strategy. Given the previously illustrated benefits of an interdisciplinary setting [8], such as a DSD or anorectal malformation clinic, these patients are ideal candidates for management within this organizational structure.

3.4. Peri-Procedural Management

When the healthcare team and patient have decided to move forward with surgical intervention for the outflow tract obstruction, there are certain anatomic considerations and patient decisions that will inform whether vaginoplasty, uterine reconnection or reconstruction, hysterectomy, or any combination are performed.

What is necessary for the long-term health and well-being of the patient? The presence of OTO and the associated surgical intervention can lead to life-altering and potentially life-threatening infection and/or urinary or gastrointestinal tract complications. For this reason, all of the goals listed below should be balanced against the short- and long-term surgical and medical risks in a comprehensive shared decision-making process.

What is the goal for sexual activity? The ability to have penetrative sexual activity may not be an immediate concern for these patients, as they often present in younger adolescence, or they may prefer different intimate activities. However, if menstrual suppression is the initial management strategy, the desire to become sexually active or have the ability to decide to do so may factor into decisions regarding the timing and type of surgical management. The goal of surgery is to create a vaginal introitus that is both large enough for menstrual egress and functional for penetrative sexual activities, should the patient desire to do so in the future.

What is the goal for fertility preservation? The fertility issue may require multiple counseling sessions and, if needed, involvement of a reproductive endocrinology and infertility (REI) specialist. REI input is helpful, as the patient's congenital and reconstructed anatomy may not allow for spontaneous conception, oocyte harvesting, embryo implantation, and/or carrying of a pregnancy to term. These considerations will help determine if uterine preservation is helpful to the patient's goals.

Several retrospective series show that, historically, patient and provider have tended towards hysterectomy to eliminate the risk of recurrent OTO, which is the concern with uterine-preserving procedures. Specific to patients with a cloacal malformation, in one older series of 22 patients, all 9 of the post-pubertal patients who presented with abdominal pain and obstruction underwent a hemi- or total hysterectomy [28]. For patients with cloacal exstrophy, 13 of the 31 individuals in one series underwent Müllerian procedures after initial reconstruction; 7 of these 13 underwent hemi- or total hysterectomy, with OTO listed as one of the indications [14]. A well-described timeline of interventions for patients with 46,XX cloacal exstrophy showed that, of 13 post-pubertal patients, 6 retained their entire uterus, 2 had hemi-hysterectomies, and the remaining 5 had total hysterectomies. Of note, the two patients with OTO both had hysterectomies [15]. Although there may be a possibility for pregnancy in these patients, when weighing the risks and benefits of recurrent OTO and need for re-operation, many patients choose hysterectomy. However, a uterine-preserving procedure should always be discussed if the patient is understanding of the risks and benefits. Clearly, patient age and maturity as well as family dynamics and consent issues are a complex part of these decisions.

Some patients may have questions regarding heritability of this condition when deciding about future fertility. Although there is currently no known genetic etiology of these conditions, and there are not enough offspring reported to see if there is a clinically significant increased risk of heritability, this would be an ideal time to involve the genetics team to help address this concern. Given the rapid pace of identification of genetic conditions with the incorporation of next-generation sequencing methods into clinical testing, it is possible that a genetic etiology might be identified in the future.

Where is the obstruction? After years of menstrual suppression, updated imaging may be necessary to redefine the OTO. Dependent upon their congenital or reconstructed anatomy, the obstruction may be just inside the introitus or more proximal. If it is a proximal obstruction, it could be related to the bowel neovagina anastomosis site or a congenital obstruction if the vagina failed to be identified at the infant evaluation. The location of the obstruction may have been elucidated from a previous MRI; however, vaginoscopy or fluoroscopy can aide in determining the optimal surgical approach.

What should the surgical approach be? Surgical creativity may be necessary when approaching these patients, and it is imperative to discuss with the patients that there are several options and that the final decision may need to be made in the operating room by the surgical team. In order to relieve the obstruction, either the native vagina needs to be brought down to the perineum, or the gap between the introitus and the native vagina or uterus needs to be bridged. There are a variety of described options and numerous considerations to accomplish this goal. Each of these different approaches has varying degrees of invasiveness and surgical risk, which is imperative to discuss and explore with the patient and their support system prior to surgical consent. This clearly highlights the need for interdisciplinary surgical care with pediatric surgery, urology, gynecology, and plastic surgery collaboration. Options for surgical intervention may include:

- Interposition with a skin graft or buccal mucosa [29];
- Small or large bowel interposition [30];
- Complex pediatric laparoscopy to mobilize the native vagina down to the perineum [31];
- Vaginal switch technique—in the presence of two hemivaginas and two hemiureteri, one hemiuterus is removed, and the associated hemivagina is tubularized with the contralateral hemivagina to lengthen the vaginal canal to the perineum [32].

3.5. Long-Term Surveillance

Recurrence of outflow obstruction is predicated on the patient having had a uterine-preserving procedure. Those who have uterine-preserving procedures must undergo regular symptom and intermittent imaging evaluations to ensure recurrence of OTO is identified early. These patients may require continued hormonal suppression to aid in dilation and treatment of possible endometriosis. If there is recurrence of OTO, we recommend repeating the management strategy outlined in this review (Table 2). All patients should follow closely with their reconstruction team and, in particular, gynecology for vaginal patency and sexual activity concerns as well as contraception, suppression for pain, and preventive health screening. If sexuality issues arise, psychology or sexual health therapists could be consulted.

For those interested in pregnancy, we recommend preconception counseling with REI, maternal fetal medicine, and the previous surgical team to create a pregnancy and delivery plan prior to conception. Cesarean delivery is likely to be recommended due to the risk to their reconstructed pelvic floor anatomy that can occur with vaginal delivery in patients with a cloacal malformation or cloacal exstrophy. These patients may have transitioned away from the surgical team; however, most tertiary care facilities will have gynecologic, urologic, and surgical specialists that will help navigate anatomic concerns surrounding pregnancy and delivery. Adult teams should not hesitate to involve their pediatric counterparts even as patients age.

4. Conclusions

Adolescent Müllerian outflow tract obstruction in patients born with a cloacal malformation or 46,XX cloacal exstrophy requires the expertise of multiple medical and surgical specialties. We strongly recommend an interdisciplinary team approach to navigate the stages of pre-obstruction education, presentation and symptom temporization, readiness assessment, peri-procedural management, and long-term surveillance. This expanded team approach should improve short- and long-term outcomes and patient satisfaction.

Author Contributions: Conceptualization, B.S.S. and M.L.D.; writing—original draft preparation, B.S.S. and M.L.D.; writing—review and editing, B.S.S., K.E.S., A.L.H., D.E.S., K.H.K., M.W.R., C.E.K., E.H.Q. and M.L.D. All authors have read and agreed to the published version of the manuscript.

Funding: This research received no external funding.

Institutional Review Board Statement: Not applicable.

Informed Consent Statement: Not applicable.

Data Availability Statement: Not applicable.

Conflicts of Interest: The authors declare no conflict of interest.

References

1. Breech, L. Gynecologic concerns in patients with anorectal malformations. *Semin. Pediatr. Surg.* **2010**, *19*, 139–145. [CrossRef] [PubMed]
2. Kapczuk, K.; Friebe, Z.; Iwaniec, K.; Kędzia, W. Obstructive Müllerian Anomalies in Menstruating Adolescent Girls: A Report of 22 Cases. *J. Pediatr. Adolesc. Gynecol.* **2018**, *31*, 252–257. [CrossRef] [PubMed]
3. Schall, K.; Parks, M.; Nemivant, S.; Hernandez, J.; Weidler, E.M. Pelvic pain in patients with complex mullerian anomalies including Mayer-Rokitansky-Kuster-Hauser syndrome (MRKH), obstructed hemi-vagina ipsilateral renal anomaly (OHVIRA), and complex cloaca. *Semin. Pediatr. Surg.* **2019**, *28*, 150842. [CrossRef] [PubMed]
4. Versteegh, H.P.; van Rooij, I.A.; Levitt, M.A.; Sloots, C.E.; Wijnen, R.M.; de Blaauw, I. Long-term follow-up of functional outcome in patients with a cloacal malformation: A systematic review. *J. Pediatr. Surg.* **2013**, *48*, 2343–2350. [CrossRef]
5. Pradhan, S.; Vilanova-Sanchez, A.; McCracken, K.A.; Reck, C.A.; Halleran, D.R.; Wood, R.J.; Levitt, M.; Hewitt, G.D. The Mullerian Black Box: Predicting and defining Mullerian anatomy in patients with cloacal abnormalities and the need for longitudinal assessment. *J. Pediatr. Surg.* **2018**, *53*, 2164–2169. [CrossRef]
6. Dietrich, J.E.; Millar, D.M.; Quint, E.H. Obstructive reproductive tract anomalies. *J. Pediatr. Adolesc. Gynecol.* **2014**, *27*, 396–402. [CrossRef]
7. Johnson, S.B. Increasing psychology's role in health research and health care. *Am. Psychol.* **2013**, *68*, 311–321. [CrossRef]
8. Lee, P.A.; Nordenström, A.; Houk, C.P.; Ahmed, S.F.; Auchus, R.; Baratz, A.; Dalke, K.B.; Liao, L.-M.; Lin-Su, K.; Looijenga, L.; et al. Global Disorders of Sex Development Update since 2006: Perceptions, Approach and Care. *Horm. Res. Paediatr.* **2016**, *85*, 158–180. [CrossRef]
9. Speck, K.E.; Arnold, M.A.; Ivancic, V.; Teitelbaum, D.H. Cloaca and hydrocolpos: Laparoscopic-, cystoscopic- and colposcopic-assisted vaginostomy tube placement. *J. Pediatr. Surg.* **2014**, *49*, 1867–1869. [CrossRef]
10. Burgu, B.; Duffy, P.G.; Cuckow, P.; Ransley, P.; Wilcox, D.T. Long-term outcome of vaginal reconstruction: Comparing techniques and timing. *J. Pediatr. Urol.* **2007**, *3*, 316–320. [CrossRef]
11. Dougherty, D.; van Leeuwen, K.D.; Sack, B.S.; Quint, E.H.; Jarboe, M.D.; Ralls, M.W. An Alternative Approach to Single-Stage Cloaca Repair: Image-Guided Anorectoplasty with Delayed Vaginoplasty. *J. Pediatr. Adolesc. Gynecol.* **2022**, *35*, 496–500. [CrossRef] [PubMed]

12. Hendren, W.H. Cloaca, the most severe degree of imperforate anus: Experience with 195 cases. *Ann. Surg.* **1998**, *228*, 331–346. [CrossRef] [PubMed]
13. Feldkamp, M.L.; Botto, L.D.; Amar, E.; Bakker, M.K.; Bermejo-Sanchez, E.; Bianca, S.; Canfield, M.A.; Castilla, E.E.; Clementi, M.; Csaky-Szunyogh, M.; et al. Cloacal exstrophy: An epidemiologic study from the International Clearinghouse for Birth Defects Surveillance and Research. *Am. J. Med. Genet. Part C Semin. Med. Genet.* **2011**, *157*, 333–343. [CrossRef] [PubMed]
14. Suson, K.D.; Preece, J.; Di Carlo, H.N.; Baradaran, N.; Gearhart, J.P. Complexities of Mullerian Anatomy in 46XX Cloacal Exstrophy Patients. *J. Pediatr. Adolesc. Gynecol.* **2016**, *29*, 424–428. [CrossRef] [PubMed]
15. Naiditch, J.A.; Radhakrishnan, J.; Chin, A.C.; Cheng, E.; Yerkes, E.; Reynolds, M. Fate of the uterus in 46XX cloacal exstrophy patients. *J. Pediatr. Surg.* **2013**, *48*, 2043–2046. [CrossRef]
16. Lund, D.P.; Hendren, W.H. Cloacal exstrophy: A 25-year experience with 50 cases. *J. Pediatr. Surg.* **2001**, *36*, 68–75. [CrossRef]
17. Siminoff, L.A.; Sandberg, D.E. Promoting Shared Decision Making in Disorders of Sex Development (DSD): Decision Aids and Support Tools. *Horm. Metab. Res.* **2015**, *47*, 335–339. [CrossRef]
18. Mizia, K.; Bennett, M.J.; Dudley, J.; Morrisey, J. Mullerian dysgenesis: A review of recent outcomes at Royal Hospital for Women. *Aust. N. Z. J. Obstet. Gynaecol.* **2006**, *46*, 29–31. [CrossRef]
19. Filipas, D.; Black, P.; Hohenfellner, R. The use of isolated caecal bowel segment in complicated vaginal reconstruction. *BJU Int.* **2000**, *85*, 715–719. [CrossRef]
20. Krege, S.; Walz, K.H.; Hauffa, B.P.; Korner, I.; Rubben, H. Long-term follow-up of female patients with congenital adrenal hyperplasia from 21-hydroxylase deficiency, with special emphasis on the results of vaginoplasty. *BJU Int.* **2000**, *86*, 253–258; discussion 258–259. [CrossRef]
21. Ugur, M.; Turan, C.; Mungan, T.; Kuşçu, E.; Şenöz, S.; Ağis, H.T.; Gökmen, O. Endometriosis in association with mullerian anomalies. *Gynecol. Obstet. Investig.* **1995**, *40*, 261–264. [CrossRef]
22. Williams, C.E.; Nakhal, R.S.; Hall-Craggs, M.A.; Wood, D.; Cutner, A.; Pattison, S.H.; Creighton, S.M. Transverse vaginal septae: Management and long-term outcomes. *BJOG Int. J. Obstet. Gynaecol.* **2014**, *121*, 1653–1658. [CrossRef]
23. Vilanova-Sanchez, A.; McCracken, K.; Halleran, D.R.; Wood, R.J.; Reck-Burneo, C.A.; Levitt, M.A.; Hewitt, G. Obstetrical Outcomes in Adult Patients Born with Complex Anorectal Malformations and Cloacal Anomalies: A Literature Review. *J. Pediatr. Adolesc. Gynecol.* **2019**, *32*, 7–14. [CrossRef]
24. Miller, R.J.; Breech, L.L. Surgical correction of vaginal anomalies. *Clin. Obstet. Gynecol.* **2008**, *51*, 223–236. [CrossRef]
25. Callens, N.; De Cuypere, G.; De Sutter, P.; Monstrey, S.; Weyers, S.; Hoebeke, P.; Cools, M. An update on surgical and non-surgical treatments for vaginal hypoplasia. *Hum. Reprod. Update* **2014**, *20*, 775–801. [CrossRef]
26. Mukherjee, B.; McCauley, E.; Hanford, R.B.; Aalsma, M.; Anderson, A.M. Psychopathology, psychosocial, gender and cognitive outcomes in patients with cloacal exstrophy. *J. Urol.* **2007**, *178*, 630–635, discussion 634–635. [CrossRef]
27. Ebert, A.; Scheuering, S.; Schott, G.; Roesch, W.H. Psychosocial and psychosexual development in childhood and adolescence within the exstrophy-epispadias complex. *J. Urol.* **2005**, *174*, 1094–1098. [CrossRef]
28. Levitt, M.A.; Stein, D.M.; Pena, A. Gynecologic concerns in the treatment of teenagers with cloaca. *J. Pediatr. Surg.* **1998**, *33*, 188–193. [CrossRef]
29. van Leeuwen, K.; Baker, L.; Grimsby, G. Autologous buccal mucosa graft for primary and secondary reconstruction of vaginal anomalies. *Semin. Pediatr. Surg.* **2019**, *28*, 150843. [CrossRef]
30. Sharma, S.; Gupta, D.K. Early vaginal replacement in cloacal malformation. *Pediatr. Surg. Int.* **2019**, *35*, 263–269. [CrossRef]
31. Demehri, F.R.; Tirrell, T.F.; Shaul, D.B.; Sydorak, R.M.; Zhong, W.; McNamara, E.R.; Borer, J.G.; Dickie, B.H. A New Approach to Cloaca: Laparoscopic Separation of the Urogenital Sinus. *J. Laparoendosc. Adv. Surg. Tech.* **2020**, *30*, 1257–1262. [CrossRef] [PubMed]
32. Bischoff, A.; Levitt, M.A.; Breech, L.; Hall, J.; Pena, A. Vaginal switch—a useful technical alternative to vaginal replacement for select cases of cloaca and urogenital sinus. *J. Pediatr. Surg.* **2013**, *48*, 363–366. [CrossRef] [PubMed]

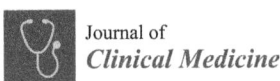

Article

Body Image and Quality of Life in Women with Congenital Adrenal Hyperplasia

Lea Tschaidse [1], Marcus Quinkler [2], Hedi Claahsen-van der Grinten [3], Anna Nordenström [4,5], Aude De Brac de la Perriere [6], Matthias K. Auer [1] and Nicole Reisch [1,*]

[1] Medizinische Klinik und Poliklinik IV, Klinikum der Universität München, LMU München, 80336 Munich, Germany; lea.tschaidse@med.uni-muenchen.de (L.T.); matthias.auer@med.uni-muenchen.de (M.K.A.)
[2] Endokrinologie Charlottenburg, 10627 Berlin, Germany; marcusquinkler@t-online.de
[3] Department of Pediatric Endocrinology, Amalia Children's Hospital, Radboud Institute for Molecular Life Sciences, Radboud University Medical Center, 6500 HB Nijmegen, The Netherlands; hedi.claahsen@radboudumc.nl
[4] Department of Women's and Children's Health, Karolinska Institutet, 171 77 Stockholm, Sweden; anna.nordenstrom@ki.se
[5] Pediatric Endocrinology Unit, Astrid Lindgren Children's Hospital, Karolinska University Hospital, 171 77 Stockholm, Sweden
[6] Hospices Civils de Lyon, 69002 Lyon, France; aude.brac@chu-lyon.fr
* Correspondence: nicole.reisch@med.uni-muenchen.de

Abstract: *Objective*: Women with congenital adrenal hyperplasia due to 21-hydroxylase deficiency (CAH) may have poor quality of life (QoL) and low satisfaction with body appearance. We investigated the influence of the patients' satisfaction with their support on their QoL and body image. *Design*: Retrospective, comparative, Europe-wide study as part of the multicenter dsd-LIFE study. *Methods*: 203 women with CAH were included in this study. We investigated the patients' QoL and body image compared to a healthy control group. The patients' satisfaction with their treatment and support in childhood and adolescence as well as in adulthood was assessed by questionnaire and its influence on the patients' body image and QoL was analyzed by multiple regression models. *Results*: Women with CAH showed worse body image and poorer physical, psychological and social QoL compared to a healthy reference population. The patients' satisfaction with professional care in the last 12 months was a significant positive predictor for all four domains of QoL (psychological, physical, social, environmental). Dissatisfaction with care in childhood and adolescence and with general support through different stages of life was a significant negative predictor for QoL and body image. *Conclusions*: These results show that women with CAH have poor QoL and body image compared to a healthy reference population. Psychosocial factors such as general and family support, and social interactions with professionals have a substantial impact on QoL and body image in adult females with CAH. This should be taken into account regarding patient care and multimodal therapy.

Keywords: 21-hydroxylase deficiency; self perception; body appearance; disorder/difference in sexual differentiation; psychosocial determinants

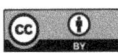

1. Introduction

Congenital adrenal hyperplasia (CAH) due to 21-hydroxylase deficiency is a rare autosomal recessive disorder characterized by impaired cortisol synthesis and in the most severe form also aldosterone synthesis. A further pathognomonic feature is adrenocorticotropic hormone (ACTH)-driven androgen excess due to reduced hypothalamo-pituitary negative feedback [1].

Care of patients with CAH can be burdensome for affected families and the social environment, as well as professional caregivers since patients face lifelong physical and psychosocial challenges due to their conditions [2,3]. In general, CAH is assumed to have greater impact on women compared to men due to unphysiological adrenal androgen excess. During female embryonic development, adrenal androgen excess causes virilization of the external genitalia in the classic form [4] that often requires genital surgery [5]. This may be associated with psychosexual challenges reflected by increased gender-atypical behavior [6], higher bi- or homosexuality [7], less frequent partnerships [8], sexual concerns and impaired satisfaction with their sex lives [9,10], as well as experienced stigmatization in sexual relations regarding their gender as well as their body appearance [11].

QoL is a complex concept for which various definitions can be found in the literature [12–15]. Since in this study QoL was assessed using a World Health Organization (WHO) questionnaire, the following definition should be noted: *"Quality of Life is defined as individuals' perceptions of their position in life in the context of the culture and value systems in which they live and in relation to their goals, expectations, standards and concerns"* [14]. The WHO concept of QoL includes four domains, which are physical, psychological, environmental and social QoL. This definition thus captures QoL as a subjective evaluation by the individual in relation to internal and external factors. This is in line with other definitions of QoL, where it is described as a multidimensional construct that is influenced by environmental and personal factors and includes both subjective and objective aspects [16].

Looking at previous research, health status [4], genotype [17] and hormonal treatment [18] were found to be important predictors for health-related QoL in CAH and in patients with disorders of sex development (DSD) in general [19]. It was also found that good social support and quality of professional care could be associated with positive outcomes in women with CAH [20]. Findings concerning the QoL in women with CAH, however, are inconsistent [4,8,21,22].

Due to adrenal androgen excess and its virilizing effect in female patients, body image is an important outcome measure in women with CAH. In the literature, body image is generally described as a multidimensional construct that contains a person's attitude towards their own body, including its perception, as well as feelings and thoughts about it [23–28]. In this context, the term body image comprises multiple categories, including body satisfaction or dissatisfaction, body acceptance and others [24,29]. Body image is influenced by various aspects, such as cognition, affect and behavior [24,25]. However, studies also show other influencing factors on body image, such as social environment, social media and beauty standards in society [30,31]. Thus, according to research, body image is influenced by both internal and external factors.

When focusing on women with CAH, studies indicate that they are less satisfied with their total body appearance [32], in particular with regard to their subjective view on the physical appearance of their genitals [17]. This seems to be influenced by surgical care, since repeated and multiple genital surgeries lead to dissatisfaction with physical appearance in patients with DSD [33], whereas other studies could not confirm this [22,34].

Although there have been studies in other areas on post-operative body image [24,35–38] some aspects are unique to this study. Women with CAH are typically operated on in childhood which is a vulnerable time [10]. In addition to this, the surgical field is a very private area and repeated examinations are uncomfortable and can lead to feelings of embarrassment among the patients. In addition, sometimes several surgical interventions are necessary [10]. Furthermore, body image in women with CAH is not only influenced by the virilized or operated genitalia, but also by other physical aspects that are caused by hyperandrogenaemia, such as a hirsutism, acne or a deeper voice [39,40]. These symptoms can persist and also affect body image, regardless of surgery.

This is the first study in CAH to investigate if and how professional and social support and quality of professional and psychological care in different stages of life influence body image and different domains of QoL, such as physical, psychological, environmental and social QoL. For this purpose, we firstly compared QoL and body image of our cohort with control groups to identify possible significant differences between these groups. Secondly, we identified important psychosocial factors in patients with CAH. Lastly, we investigated the influence of these psychosocial and other factors on QoL and body image of our patients and identified significant positive and negative predictors for these outcome variables.

2. Material and Methods
2.1. Study Design

The data from this study were collected within the "dsd-LIFE" study, a European multicenter cross-sectional study funded by the European Commission (7th Framework Program, FP7). From February 2014 to September 2015 participants were recruited in 14 specialized clinical centers in 6 countries (France ($n = 4$), Germany ($n = 4$), Poland ($n = 2$), the Netherlands ($n = 2$), Sweden ($n = 1$) and the United Kingdom ($n = 1$)). Patients were enrolled if they had a medically confirmed clinical or genetic diagnosis of DSD, were at least 16 years of age, and presented to a study center at least once during the course of the study. Patients who did not fulfill the diagnostic criteria or could not consent nor answer the questionnaire by themselves, were excluded. A total of 1040 patients met the inclusion criteria and of these, 203 were females diagnosed with CAH and were therefore included in the study. Ethical approval was received for each study center and all participants gave written informed consent. The study consisted of 2 parts: the first part took place at the respective study center and consisted of a medical interview and an optional medical examination; the second part consisted of a digital patient-reported outcome (PRO) questionnaire and was filled out online. If necessary, a paper pencil form was available. All medical data were pseudonymized and reviewed regarding accuracy of statement. Further information on the theoretical and methodological background of the study can be found elsewhere [41].

Sociodemographic data were collected using the European Social Survey (ESS Round 7, 2015) as well as self-constructed items. The educational status of the participants was measured by the ES-ISCED as a part of the ESS. It categorizes education in "low" (ESISCED 1–2), "middle" (ESISCED 3–5) and "high" (ESISCED 6–7) [18].

To assess QoL the WHOQOL-BREF Questionnaire was used. It consists of 24 items describing 4 different domains of QoL (physical, psychological, environmental, social), with 3 to 8 items per domain. All items are answered on a 5-Point Likert Scale. For each domain 2 different scales can be used with scores either ranging from 0–100 or from 4–20, with higher scores indicating a higher QoL. Both scales can be converted into each other [14].

To measure the participants' body image, the Body image scale (BIS) was used. The BIS is intended to not only measure the perception about one's own body but also the feeling about this perception. It consists of questions about 30 body features, which the participants have to rate on a 5-point scale of satisfaction (1 = very satisfied to 5 = very dissatisfied). A total of 27 body features are gender neutral, 3 are gender-related, concerning the internal and external genitals. In this study, the female items were included in the analysis. Eventually, the items' scores were added up and divided by the number of items, which led to a final mean score ranging from 1 to 5. A higher score indicates higher dissatisfaction with appearance of the own body [27].

Concerning the 4 domains of QoL a reference popualtion was used consisting of 2055 individuals, 927 males and 1128 females [42]. Of these, 250 were young adults aged between 18 and 25 years, and 393 were elderly people who were 66 years and older [42]. For body image, a reference population was used that included 57 female university students aged between 19 and 35 years [36].

As the aim of the study was to assess psychosocial determinants, several domains of the PRO Questionnaire were included, which displayed the participants' satisfaction with their treatment and support in childhood, adolescence, adulthood resepectively. Therefore, the following domains were included in the analysis: "Diagnosis and Disclosure", "Your treatment in childhood/adolescence", "Psychological care and general support in childhood/adolescence", "Satisfaction with care", and "Satisfaction with psychological and general support in adulthood". These categories asked the patients about whether information about the condition, hormone therapy and surgical procedures were given fully and in a sensitive and understandable way during childhood and adolescence. Furthermore, whether the patients were properly informed about treatment options, including risks and side effects, and whether they were satisfied the way physical examinations took place and the doctors' behavior and knowledge of childhood, adolescence and adulthood. Additionally, it was asked if the patients were satisfied with general support from parents, friends, partners and doctors in childhood, adolescence and adulthood. The items of these categories were either self-constructed or taken from the Child Health Care–Satisfaction, Utilization and Needs (CHC-SUN9) Questionnaire, as well as the Customer Satisfaction Questionnaire (CSQ-4). Most of the items were to be answered on a 4- to 5-point scale.

2.2. Statistical Analysis

In order to compare body image and QoL of women with CAH to a healthy reference population Welch's tests were conducted as recommended [43]. The Bonferroni–Holm correction was used for multiple testing.

To assess psychosocial determinants, 38 items were included in the statistical analysis. As these items were not part of a validated instrument but either self-constructed or taken from different measuring instruments, they could not be summed up by predetermined criteria. Therefore, to reduce data for further analysis, an explorative factor analysis was performed. The data's eligibility for a factor analysis was tested as recommended [44] and based on the results a principal component analysis with oblique promax rotation was carried out extracting 2 factors. In total, the 2 factors explained 45.79% of the variance, factor I with an eigenvalue of 12.04 explained 31.68% and factor II with an eigenvalue of 5.36 explained an additional 14.12%.

To investigate the impact of the psychosocial determinants on the participants' body images and the different domains of QoL, multiple linear regression models were built for each outcome variable (BIS-Score, physical QoL, psychological QoL, environmental QoL, social QoL). As recent studies showed an influence of age, country and education on patients living with DSD or CAH in particular [19,45], we included these variables in the analysis. Given that previous research has demonstrated that genital surgery has a negative impact on satisfaction of total body appearance in patients with CAH [32] and could influence QoL in patients with DSD [8], it was included in the analysis, as was Body-Mass-Index (BMI) since obesity is a common problem in women with CAH and seems to affect QoL negatively [4]. Ultimately, age at diagnosis was added as this is related to the severity of CAH [10]. The analysis was conducted by using the method of block-wise inclusion.

For the statistical analysis, IBM SPSS Statistics 26.0 was used. Missing values were replaced by the mean value of the respective variable. A significance level of $\alpha = 0.05$ was determined for the statistical analysis of this study.

3. Results

3.1. Patient Characteristics

The final study population consisted of 203 female patients with CAH. The largest part of the study population was recruited in Germany ($n = 86$, 42.36%), followed by France ($n = 52$, 25.62%), the Netherlands ($n = 22$, 10.84%), the United Kingdom ($n = 18$, 8.87%), Poland ($n = 14$, 6.90%) and Sweden ($n = 11$, 5.42%). Further details of the study population are displayed in Table 1.

Table 1. General characteristics.

	n	Total n	%
Number of patients		203	
Country		203	
Germany	86		42.36
France	52		25.62

Table 1. Cont.

		n	Total n	%
Netherlands		22		10.84
Poland		14		6.90
Sweden		11		5.42
United Kingdom		18		8.87
Education			203	
Low (ESISCED 1–2)		40		19.70
Middle (ESISCED 3–5)		97		47.78
High (ESISCED 6–7)		48		23.65
Unknown		18		8.87
Median age at assessment (min–max) in years	30.28 (15.0–68.0)		203	
Age at diagnosis			203	
Before birth		14		6.90
At birth (0–1 month)		109		53.69
Infancy (1 month–3 years)		33		16.26
Childhood (4–12 years)		15		7.39
Adolescence (13–17 years)		10		4.93
Adulthood ($\geq$18 years)		20		9.85
Unknown		2		0.99
Median BMI at assessment (min–max)	26.45 (15.60–46.40)		199	
Genital surgery			203	
Yes		160		78.82
No		42		20.69
Unknown		1		0.49

Description of the study population: Minimum (min); Maximum (max); Body mass index (BMI).

3.2. Body Image and QoL in Women with CAH

The basic descriptive statistics of the outcome variables can be seen in Table 2. All four domains of QoL and the BIS-Score were compared to reference populations. While women with CAH showed a significantly poorer body image, physical, psychological and social QoL, they showed significantly better environmental QoL compared to controls. Post-hoc effect size Cohen's d was analyzed using G*Power, showing small to medium effect sizes [46]. The results can be seen in Table 3.

Table 2. Body image and QoL outcomes.

Outcome Variable			n = 203		
	M	SD	Range	Min	Max
BIS-Score	2.5	0.7	4.0	1.0	5.0
Physical QoL					
Range 0–100	68.7	18.8	82.1	17.9	100.0
Range 4–20	15.0	3.0	13.1	6.9	20.0
Psychological QoL					

Table 2. Cont.

Outcome Variable			n = 203		
	M	SD	Range	Min	Max
Range 0–100	66.0	18.3	87.5	12.5	100.0
Range 4–20	14.6	2.9	14.0	6.0	20.0
Environmental QoL					
Range 0–100	74.6	15.5	75.0	25.0	100.0
Range 4–20	15.9	2.5	12.0	8.0	20.0
Social QoL					
Range 0–100	64.7	20.8	91.7	8.3	100.0
Range 4–20	14.4	3.3	14.7	5.3	20.0

Description of the outcome variables with mean score (M), standard deviation (SD), range, minimum (Min) and maximum (Max). Body image scale (BIS). The scores for domains of quality of life (QoL) are depicted with range 0–100 as well as 4–20.

Table 3. Comparison of outcome variables of women with CAH and healthy reference populations.

Variable	CAH Group			Reference Group			df	t	p	d
	n	M	SD	n	M	SD				
BIS-Score	203	2.5	0.7	57	2.4	0.3	196	2.38	0.018	0.19
Physical QoL	203	68.7	18.8	2052	76.9	17.7	239	−5.96	<0.001	0.45
Psych. QoL	203	66.0	18.3	2055	74.0	15.7	232	−6.01	<0.001	0.47
Envir. QoL	203	74.6	15.5	2053	70.4	14.2	237	3.71	<0.001	0.28
Social QoL	203	64.7	20.8	2048	71.8	18.5	235	−4.68	<0.001	0.36

Display of Body image scale (BIS)-Score and the 4 domains of quality of life (QoL) of the study population and reference populations [27,28]. Psych. QoL describes psychological QoL and Envir. QoL describes environmental QoL. Congenital adrenal hyperplasia (CAH). Description of the outcome variables with mean score (M), standard deviation (SD).

3.3. Correlation between QoL Dimensions and BIS-Score

A correlation matrix for the four domains of QoL and the BIS-Score was built and is presented in Table 4. As BIS-Sore was the only variable that met the criteria for normal distribution Spearman's rho was used. All four dimensions of QoL intercorrelated significantly ($p < 0.001$) with a positive correlation coefficient ranging from $r = 0.43$ to $r = 0.67$. The BIS-Score correlated significantly ($p < 0.001$) with all four domains of QoL with a negative correlation coefficient ranging from $r = -0.41$ to $r = -0.56$. This indicates that good QoL in one domain is associated with good QoL in the other domains as well as good body image.

Table 4. Correlation matrix of the outcome variables.

	BIS-Score	Physical QoL	Psych. QoL	Envir. QoL	Social QoL
BIS-Score					
Physical QoL	−0.42				
Psych. QoL	−0.56	0.67			
Envir. QoL	−0.41	0.62	0.67		
Social QoL	−4.2	0.43	0.60	0.53	

Body image scale (BIS) and quality of life (QoL). Psych. QoL describes psychological QoL and Envir. QoL describes environmental QoL. All correlations were significant with a p-value < 0.001.

3.4. Psychosocial Determinants in Women with CAH

The factor analysis revealed two psychosocial factors. Factor I contained all items of the categories "Diagnosis and Disclosure", "Your treatment in childhood and adolescence", "Psychological care and general support in childhood and adolescence" included in the analysis and three items of the category "Satisfaction with psychological and general support in adulthood". These items loading on factor I can be summarized as "Dissatisfaction with care in childhood and adolescence and with general support through different stages of life".

Factor II contained all items of the category "Satisfaction with care in the last 12 months" and one item of the category "Satisfaction with psychological and general support in adulthood". The items loading on factor II can be summarized as "Satisfaction with professional care in the last 12 months".

3.5. Influence of Psychosocial Determinants on Body Image and QoL

The results for the multiple regression models with significant predictors for body image (BIS-Score) and the different domains of QoL are depicted in Table 5. Our linear regression models explained 13% of variance of body image as well as 38% (physical QoL), 34% (psychological QoL), 33% (environmental QoL) and 23% (social QoL) of variance of the different domains of QoL. Both psychosocial factors were included in the multiple regression models. Factor I "Dissatisfaction with care in childhood and adolescence and with general support through different stages of life" was a significant positive predictor of the BIS-Score (i.e., lower body image) and a significant negative predictor of all four domains of QoL. Factor II "Satisfaction with professional care in the last 12 months", was a significant positive predictor of all four domains of QoL but was not a significant predictor of the BIS-Score.

Table 5. Linear Regression models of the outcome variables.

Outcome Variable	Predictor Variable	β	t	p	Adj. R^2	R^2
BIS-Score						
	Country				0.0	0.03
	Sweden	−0.15	−2.04	0.043		
	Educational level				0.01	0.05
	High	−0.18	−2.12	0.036		
	BMI	0.22	3.01	0.003	0.04	0.08
	Psychosocial Factor I	0.24	3.03	0.003	0.12	0.19
Physical QoL						
	Country				0.1	0.13
	France	−0.36	−5.66	<0.001		
	UK	−0.19	−3.15	0.002		
	Educational level				0.17	0.21
	Middle	0.23	3.33	0.001		
	High	0.33	4.54	<0.001		
	BMI	−0.13	−2.19	0.03	0.18	0.21
	Age at diagnosis					
	Infancy	0.2	2.07	0.04	0.22	0.28
	Psychosocial Factor I	−0.27	−3.98	<0.001	0.34	0.39
	Psychosocial Factor II	0.25	3.83	<0.001	0.38	0.43

Table 5. Cont.

Outcome Variable	Predictor Variable	β	t	p	Adj. R^2	R^2
Psych. QoL						
	Country				0.02	0.05
	France	−0.14	−2.19	0.03		
	Poland	−0.13	−2.13	0.035		
	UK	−0.15	−2.3	0.022		
	Educational level				0.03	0.07
	High	0.15	2.0	0.047		
	Psychosocial Factor I	−0.28	−3.98	<0.001	0.29	0.23
	Psychosocial Factor II	0.38	5.59	<0.001	0.34	0.4
Envir. QoL						
	Country				0.01	0.04
	France	−0.27	−4.16	<0.001		
	Educational level				0.05	0.08
	Middle	0.18	2.5	0.013		
	High	0.22	2.97	0.003		
	Psychosocial Factor I	−0.29	−4.09	<0.001	0.22	0.28
	Psychosocial Factor II	0.38	5.55	<0.001	0.33	0.39
Social QoL						
	Educational level				0.07	0.11
	High	0.28	3.43	0.001		
	Psychosocial Factor I	−0.23	−3.01	0.003	0.16	0.23
	Psychosocial Factor II	0.31	4.17	<0.001	0.23	0.29

Displayed are significant predictors of the outcome variables with β, t-value, p-value, adjusted R^2, R^2. Body image scale (BIS) and quality of life (QoL). Psych. QoL describes psychological QoL and Envir. QoL describes environmental QoL. Body mass index (BMI).

4. Discussion

Our results show that women with CAH have worse body image and poorer physical, psychological and social QoL compared to a healthy reference population. In our model, a better body image was predicted by a high level of education, whilst a higher BMI and dissatisfaction with care and general support predicted a worse body image. Furthermore, the study shows that psychosocial factors such as general and family support or social interaction with professionals have a substantial impact on QoL and body image in adult women with CAH. More precisely, it was shown that satisfaction with professional care in the last 12 months has a great impact on women's QoL, whereas care in childhood and adolescence and social support additionally impact on body image.

Interestingly, our regression model identified general support and satisfaction with professional care in childhood and adolescence as an influencing factor for body image in women with CAH but not satisfaction with professional care in the last 12 months. These findings are consistent with a study showing that negative experience with parental care during childhood was associated with body insecurity and dissatisfaction with physical appearance later in life in patients with DSD [33]. Positive experience with parental care, on the other hand, was associated with a higher feeling of body attractiveness [33]. It can be speculated that developing a coping ability in childhood and adolescence is an underlying mechanism of these findings. Parental support from health care practitioners may be an important factor resulting in more positive parental care and better body image in their daughters affected by CAH. Additionally, we found that a higher BMI is associated with worse body image. This is consistent with previous studies, both for healthy women [31], and for women with other chronic conditions [47].

Regarding QoL, we found that women with CAH have higher environmental QoL compared to a healthy reference population [42] whilst having lower physical, psychological and social QoL. This is consistent with findings that show decreased QoL in women with DSD, especially in women with CAH, 46,XX and 46,XY- virilized females, using the QoL-AGHDA Questionnaire [8]. It also suggests that a higher degree of virilisation could be associated with a poorer QoL. The UKChase study examining 203 male and female patients with CAH also found decreased QoL across all eight domains of the SF-36 questionnaire [4], as did a study from Norway [48]. However, high doses of glucocorticoids might worsen QoL as well, probably through metabolic changes (e.g., obesity), suppression of the gonadal axis and neuropsychological changes, e.g observed in patients with Cushing's syndrome. Reduction in high doses of glucocorticoids seems to improve QoL in CAH patients [49].

As the domain social QoL contains aspects of interpersonal relationships and sexual activity [14] our findings are in line with research showing less experience with love and sexual relationships in patients with DSD [50] and decreased satisfaction with sex life in women with CAH [10].

Our regression models identified both psychosocial factors, i.e., satisfaction with professional care in the last 12 months as well as dissatisfaction with care in childhood and adolescence and with general support through different stages of life as significant predictors for the patients' QoL. Satisfaction with professional care in the last 12 months was found to be a strong positive predictor for all four domains of QoL. Previous research confirms that the degree of satisfaction with professional care is directly associated with health-related QoL in patients with DSD [51]. Dissatisfaction with care in childhood and adolescence and general support at any stage of life, on the other hand, is an important negative predictor for the outcome of women with CAH. We found that it is associated with lower WHOQOL-BREF scores in all four domains, indicating lower QoL. In general, it was shown that children with CAH have an impaired health-related QoL compared to a healthy control group [52], which could negatively influence QoL later in life.

It has to be emphasized that only 17.2% of the participants in our study received psychological support in childhood and adolescence and the same magnitude (18.7%) in adulthood, not allowing further analysis. In itself, however, this is a remarkable and worrying result, as patients with DSD showed a higher frequency of psychological and psychiatric counselling when experiencing severe problems [8]. A study investigating psychological counselling of 110 adults with DSD showed that about one fifth of patients reported that they had never been offered psychological counselling but would have needed it, resulting in the lowest level of satisfaction with care [52]. These findings emphasize the patients' wishes and need for such care which medical staff should keep in mind while treating these patients throughout their lifetime.

In our study population, higher educational levels were associated with a better outcome in all four domains of QoL. This is in line with findings regarding physical and health-related QoL in patients with chronic diseases as well as in women with breast cancer [53,54]. In contrast, higher BMI was a negative predictor for physical QoL, which was expected, as obese women in general report lower physical QoL compared to non-obese women [55]. This is of particular interest as obesity is a common and at least in part treatment-related challenge in women with CAH [4,56]. Concerning age at diagnosis, early diagnosis was positively associated with physical QoL. Previous research demonstrated that the timing of diagnosis is associated with the severity of CAH [10] and therefore predicts clinical symptoms [57]. Hence, one explanation for this result could be that CAH forms that are diagnosed at birth are mostly more severe than those diagnosed at infancy and have a greater negative impact on physical health [58]. Lastly, genital surgery was neither a significant predictor for body image nor for the different domains of QoL. This is unexpected as research so far indicates that QoL and satisfaction with body appearance are affected by genital surgery [17]. However, these findings could be explained with the median age of about 30 years of the study sample, which is rather young. As surgical indications and procedures have evolved over the last decades, recent findings indicate that the surgical outcome for female patients with CAH has improved [59].

To our knowledge this study is the first investigating the influence of perceived quality of professional and general support on QoL and body image in women with CAH. However, this study also has several limitations. In this work, the four domains of QoL and the body image using BIS score were treated as independent endpoints. Other studies suggest that this could not be the case. A study that examined 581 women with breast cancer using the WHOQOL-BREF and a Body Image Scale for cancer patients [60] showed that the BIS score was a significant predictor for all four domains of QoL in the study population rather than an outcome variable itself [54]. Further research emphasizes these findings as it was shown that body image dissatisfaction is a negative predictor for physical and psychological health related QoL in a healthy study sample [61]. Another limitation is that no standardized instrument was used to assess psychosocial determinants but mainly self-constructed items. Many aspects were subjective and asked retrospectively which could lead to a bias caused by the participants' current state of mind.

5. Conclusions

Our results underline the importance of professional and social support for body image outcomes in this patient cohort. Interestingly, this does not seem to be limited to adult life; perceived support in childhood and adolescence also significantly influences body image later in life. This should be taken into account in the lifelong care of these patients, as their possible body image issues should already be addressed during care in childhood and adolescence. Professional caregivers and the social environment need to be educated in this regard. This is particularly important as the literature has shown the far-reaching effects of positive and negative body images.

QoL could also be predicted, among other things, by satisfaction with general support and professional care, making it a crucial factor. Therefore, in order to provide good professional support for patients with this rare disease, care should be provided at specialized centers. The goal should be a multimodal therapy concept in which different disciplines cooperate in caring for the patients. This could also address the current issue of clearly insufficient psychological support in patients with CAH that we found in our cohort. There is an urgent need for psychological counselling and therefore support should be offered repeatedly to all patients and families with children with CAH.

Author Contributions: Conceptualization, M.Q., H.C.-v.d.G., A.N., A.D.B.d.l.P. and N.R.; validation, M.K.A. and N.R.; formal analysis, L.T.; investigation, M.Q., H.C.-v.d.G., A.N., A.D.B.d.l.P. and N.R.; data curation, M.Q., H.C.-v.d.G., A.N., A.D.B.d.l.P. and N.R.; writing—original draft preparation, L.T. and N.R.; writing—review and editing, M.Q., H.C.-v.d.G., A.N., A.D.B.d.l.P. and M.K.A.; visualization, L.T., M.K.A. and N.R.; supervision, N.R.; funding acquisition, M.Q., H.C.-v.d.G., A.N., A.D.B.d.l.P. and N.R. All authors have read and agreed to the published version of the manuscript.

Funding: This work was supported by the European Union Seventh Framework Programme (grant 305373 [FP7/2007–2013]) and the Deutsche Forschungsgemeinschaft (Heisenberg Professorship 325768017 to NR and Projektnummer: 314061271-TRR205 to N.R.).

Institutional Review Board Statement: Ethical approval as appropriate to each country was obtained (ethical approval of the Ethikkommission 2 am Campus Virchow-Klinikum, University Medicine Charité Berlin, Berlin Germany, EA2/069/13).

Informed Consent Statement: Written informed consent was obtained from all subjects involved in this study.

Data Availability Statement: The data presented in this study are available on reasonable request from the corresponding author.

Acknowledgments: We thank all participants of the DSD-life study. **The dsd-LIFE Group:** Birgit Köhler, Berlin, Germany; Peggy Cohen-Kettenis and Annelou de Vries, Amsterdam, the Netherlands; Wiebke Arlt, Birmingham, United Kingdom; Claudia Wiesemann, Göttingen, Germany; Jolanta Slowikowska-Hilczer, Łódź, Poland; Aude Brac de la Perrière, Lyon, France; Charles Sultan and Francoise Paris, Montpellier, France; Claire Bouvattier, Paris, France; Ute Thyen, Lübeck, Germany; Nicole Reisch, Munich, Germany; Annette Richter-Unruh, Münster, Germany; Hedi Claahsen-van der Grinten, Nijmegen, the Netherlands; Anna Nordenström, Stockholm, Sweden; Catherine Pienkowski, Toulouse, France; and Maria Szarras-Czapnik, Warsaw, Poland.

Conflicts of Interest: All authors declare no conflict of interest. The funding sources had no role in the design of the study; collection, analysis, and interpretation of the data; writing the report; or in the decision to submit the article for publication.

References

1. El-Maouche, D.; Arlt, W.; Merke, D.P. Congenital adrenal hyperplasia. *Lancet* **2017**, *390*, 2194–2210. [CrossRef]
2. Reisch, N. Review of Health Problems in Adult Patients with Classic Congenital Adrenal Hyperplasia due to 21-Hydroxylase Deficiency. *Exp. Clin. Endocrinol. Diabetes* **2019**, *127*, 171. [CrossRef] [PubMed]
3. Tschaidse, L.; Quitter, F.; Hübner, A.; Reisch, N. [Long-term morbidity in congenital adrenal hyperplasia]. *Internist* **2022**, *63*, 43–50. [CrossRef] [PubMed]
4. Arlt, W.; Willis, D.S.; Wild, S.H.; Krone, N.; Doherty, E.J.; Hahner, S.; Han, T.; Carroll, P.V.; Conway, G.S.; Rees, A.; et al. Health Status of Adults with Congenital Adrenal Hyperplasia: A Cohort Study of 203 Patients. *J. Clin. Endocrinol. Metab.* **2010**, *95*, 5110–5121. [CrossRef] [PubMed]
5. Nordenström, A. Adult women with 21-hydroxylase deficient congenital adrenal hyperplasia, surgical and psychological aspects. *Curr. Opin. Pediatr.* **2011**, *23*, 436–442. [CrossRef] [PubMed]
6. Frisen, L.; Nordenstrom, A.; Falhammar, H.; Filipsson, H.; Holmdahl, G.; Janson, P.O.; Thoren, M.; Hagenfeldt, K.; Moller, A.; Nordenskjold, A. Gender role behavior, sexuality, and psychosocial adaptation in women with congenital adrenal hyperplasia due to CYP21A2 deficiency. *J. Clin. Endocrinol. Metab.* **2009**, *94*, 3432–3439. [CrossRef] [PubMed]
7. Meyer-Bahlburg, H.F.L.; Dolezal, C.; Baker, S.W.; New, M.I. Sexual Orientation in Women with Classical or Non-classical Congenital Adrenal Hyperplasia as a Function of Degree of Prenatal Androgen Excess. *Arch. Sex. Behav.* **2008**, *37*, 85–99. [CrossRef]
8. Johannsen, T.H.; Ripa, C.P.L.; Mortensen, E.L.; Main, K.M. Quality of life in 70 women with disorders of sex development. *Eur. J. Endocrinol.* **2006**, *155*, 877–885. [CrossRef] [PubMed]
9. Wisniewski, A.B.; Migeon, C.J.; Malouf, M.A.; Gearhart, J.P. Psychosexual Outcome in Women Affected by Congenital Adrenal Hyperplasia Due To 21-Hydroxylase Deficiency. *J. Urol.* **2004**, *171*, 2497–2501. [CrossRef]
10. Nordenström, A.; Frisén, L.; Falhammar, H.; Filipsson, H.; Holmdahl, G.; Janson, P.O.; Thorén, M.; Hagenfeldt, K.; Nordenskjöld, A. Sexual Function and Surgical Outcome in Women with Congenital Adrenal Hyperplasia Due to *CYP21A2* Deficiency: Clinical Perspective and the Patients' Perception. *J. Clin. Endocrinol. Metab.* **2010**, *95*, 3633–3640. [CrossRef]
11. Meyer-Bahlburg, H.F.L.; Khuri, J.; Reyes-Portillo, J.; Ehrhardt, A.A.; New, M.I. Stigma Associated with Classical Congenital Adrenal Hyperplasia in Women's Sexual Lives. *Arch. Sex. Behav.* **2018**, *47*, 943–951. [CrossRef] [PubMed]
12. Moons, P.; Budts, W.; De Geest, S. Critique on the conceptualisation of quality of life: A review and evaluation of different conceptual approaches. *Int. J. Nurs. Stud.* **2006**, *43*, 891–901. [CrossRef] [PubMed]
13. Post, M. Definitions of Quality of Life: What Has Happened and How to Move On. *Top. Spinal Cord Inj. Rehabil.* **2014**, *20*, 167–180. [CrossRef] [PubMed]
14. The WHOQOL Group. Development of the World Health Organization WHOQOL-BREF quality of life assessment. The WHOQOL Group. *Psychol. Med.* **1998**, *28*, 551–558. [CrossRef]
15. Karimi, M.; Brazier, J. Health, Health-Related Quality of Life, and Quality of Life: What is the Difference? *Pharmacoeconomics* **2016**, *34*, 645–649. [CrossRef]
16. Cummins, R.A. Moving from the quality of life concept to a theory. *J. Intellect. Disabil. Res.* **2005**, *49*, 699–706. [CrossRef]
17. Nordenskjöld, A.; Holmdahl, G.; Frisén, L.; Falhammar, H.; Filipsson, H.; Thorén, M.; Janson, P.O.; Hagenfeldt, K. Type of Mutation and Surgical Procedure Affect Long-Term Quality of Life for Women with Congenital Adrenal Hyperplasia. *J. Clin. Endocrinol. Metab.* **2008**, *93*, 380–386. [CrossRef]
18. Han, T.; Krone, N.; Willis, D.S.; Conway, G.S.; Hahner, S.; Rees, D.A.; Stimson, R.H.; Walker, B.R.; Arlt, W.; Ross, R.J. Quality of life in adults with congenital adrenal hyperplasia relates to glucocorticoid treatment, adiposity and insulin resistance: United Kingdom Congenital adrenal Hyperplasia Adult Study Executive (CaHASE). *Eur. J. Endocrinol.* **2013**, *168*, 887–893. [CrossRef]
19. Rapp, M.; Mueller-Godeffroy, E.; Lee, P.; Roehle, R.; Kreukels, B.P.C.; Köhler, B.; Nordenström, A.; Bouvattier, C.; Thyen, U.; dsd-LIFE Group. Multicentre cross-sectional clinical evaluation study about quality of life in adults with disorders/differences of sex development (DSD) compared to country specific reference populations (dsd-LIFE). *Heal. Qual. Life Outcomes* **2018**, *16*, 54. [CrossRef] [PubMed]

20. Kanhere, M.; Fuqua, J.; Rink, R.; Houk, C.; Mauger, D.; Lee, P.A. Psychosexual development and quality of life outcomes in females with congenital adrenal hyperplasia. *Int. J. Pediatr. Endocrinol.* **2015**, *2015*, 21. [CrossRef]
21. Jaaskelainen, J.; Voutilainen, R. Long-term outcome of classical 21-hydroxylase deficiency: Diagnosis, complications and quality of life. *Acta Paediatr.* **2000**, *89*, 183–187. [CrossRef] [PubMed]
22. Reisch, N.; Hahner, S.; Bleicken, B.; Flade, L.; Gil, F.P.; Loeffler, M.; Ventz, M.; Hinz, A.; Beuschlein, F.; Allolio, B.; et al. Quality of life is less impaired in adults with congenital adrenal hyperplasia because of 21-hydroxylase deficiency than in patients with primary adrenal insufficiency. *Clin. Endocrinol.* **2011**, *74*, 166–173. [CrossRef] [PubMed]
23. Grogan, S. Body image and health: Contemporary perspectives. *J. Health Psychol.* **2006**, *11*, 523–530. [CrossRef] [PubMed]
24. Ivezaj, V.; Grilo, C.M. The complexity of body image following bariatric surgery: A systematic review of the literature. *Obes. Rev.* **2018**, *19*, 1116–1140. [CrossRef] [PubMed]
25. Lydecker, J.A.; White, M.A.; Grilo, C.M. Form and formulation: Examining the distinctiveness of body image constructs in treatment-seeking patients with binge-eating disorder. *J. Consult. Clin. Psychol.* **2017**, *85*, 1095–1103. [CrossRef] [PubMed]
26. Baker, C.; Wertheim, E.H. Body Image: A Handbook of Theory, Research, and Clinical Practice, edited by Thomas, F. Cash and Thomas Pruzinsky, New York: Guilford Press, 2002, 530 pages, $60.00. *Eat. Disord.* **2003**, *11*, 247–248. [CrossRef]
27. Lindgren, T.W.; Pauly, I.B. A body image scale for evaluating transsexuals. *Arch. Sex. Behav.* **1975**, *4*, 639–656. [CrossRef]
28. McComb, J.; Massey-Stokes, M. Body image concerns throughout the lifespan. In *The Active Female*; Springer: New York, NY, USA, 2014; pp. 3–24.
29. Wallis, K.; Prichard, I.; Hart, L.; Yager, Z. The Body Confident Mums challenge: A feasibility trial and qualitative evaluation of a body acceptance program delivered to mothers using Facebook. *BMC Public Health* **2021**, *21*, 1052. [CrossRef]
30. Skouteris, H.; Carr, R.; Wertheim, E.H.; Paxton, S.J.; Duncombe, D. A prospective study of factors that lead to body dissatisfaction during pregnancy. *Body Image* **2005**, *2*, 347–361. [CrossRef]
31. Hardit, S.K.; Hannum, J.W. Attachment, the tripartite influence model, and the development of body dissatisfaction. *Body Image* **2012**, *9*, 469–475. [CrossRef]
32. Stikkelbroeck, N.M.; Beerendonk, C.C.; Willemsen, W.N.; Schreuders-Bais, C.; Feitz, W.F.; Rieu, P.N.; Hermus, A.R.; Otten, B.J. The long term outcome of feminizing genital surgery for congenital adrenal hyperplasia: Anatomical, functional and cosmetic outcomes, psychosexual development, and satisfaction in adult female patients. *J. Pediatr. Adolesc. Gynecol.* **2003**, *16*, 289–296. [CrossRef]
33. Schweizer, K.; Brunner, F.; Gedrose, B.; Handford, C.; Richter-Appelt, H. Coping With Diverse Sex Development: Treatment Experiences and Psychosocial Support During Childhood and Adolescence and Adult Well-Being. *J. Pediatr. Psychol.* **2017**, *42*, jsw058–519. [CrossRef] [PubMed]
34. Zucker, K.J.; Bradley, S.J.; Oliver, G.; Blake, J.; Fleming, S.; Hood, J. Self-Reported Sexual Arousability in Women with Congenital Adrenal Hyperplasia. *J. Sex Marital Ther.* **2004**, *30*, 343–355. [CrossRef] [PubMed]
35. Bertoletti, J.; Aparicio, M.J.G.; Bordignon, S.; Trentini, C.M. Body Image and Bariatric Surgery: A Systematic Review of Literature. *Bariatr. Surg. Pract. Patient Care* **2018**, *14*, 81–92. [CrossRef]
36. Van de Grift, T.C.; Kreukels, B.P.; Elfering, L.; Özer, M.; Bouman, M.-B.; Buncamper, M.E.; Smit, J.M.; Mullender, M.G. Body Image in Transmen: Multidimensional Measurement and the Effects of Mastectomy. *J. Sex. Med.* **2016**, *13*, 1778–1786. [CrossRef]
37. Song, L.; Pang, Y.; Zhang, J.; Tang, L. Body image in colorectal cancer patients: A longitudinal study. *Psycho-Oncol.* **2021**, *30*, 1339–1346. [CrossRef]
38. Shorka, D.; Yemini, N.; Ben Shushan, G.; Tokar, L.; Benbenishty, J.; Woloski-Wruble, A. Body image and scar assessment: A longitudinal cohort analysis of cardiothoracic, neurosurgery and urology patients. *J. Clin. Nurs.* **2021**. [CrossRef]
39. Nordenström, A.; Falhammar, H. Management of Endocrine Disease: Diagnosis and management of the patient with non-classic CAH due to 21-hydroxylase deficiency. *Eur. J. Endocrinol.* **2019**, *180*, R127–R145. [CrossRef]
40. Nygren, U.; Södersten, M.; Falhammar, H.; Thorén, M.; Hagenfeldt, K.; Nordenskjöld, A. Voice characteristics in women with congenital adrenal hyperplasia due to 21-hydroxylase deficiency. *Clin. Endocrinol.* **2009**, *70*, 18–25. [CrossRef]
41. Röhle, R.; Gehrmann, K.; Szarras-Czapnik, M.; der Grinten, H.C.-V.; Pienkowski, C.; Bouvattier, C.; Cohen-Kettenis, P.; Nordenström, A.; Thyen, U.; dsd-LIFE group. Participation of adults with disorders/differences of sex development (DSD) in the clinical study DSD-LIFE: Design, methodology, recruitment, data quality and study population. *BMC Endocr. Disord.* **2017**, *17*, 52. [CrossRef]
42. Angermeyer, M.; Kilian, R.; Matschinger, H. *WHOQOL–100 und WHOQOL–BREF. Handbuch für die Deutschsprachige Version der WHO Instrumente zur Erfassung der Lebensqualität*; Hogrefe: Göttingen, Germany, 2000.
43. Rasch, D.; Kubinger, K.D.; Moder, K. The two-sample *t*-test: Pre-testing its assumptions does not pay off. *Stat. Pap.* **2011**, *52*, 219–231. [CrossRef]
44. Bühner, M. *Einführung in die Test- und Fragebogenkonstruktion*, 3rd ed.; Pearson Studium: Munich, Germany, 2008. [CrossRef]
45. Strandqvist, A.; Falhammar, H.; Lichtenstein, P.; Hirschberg, A.L.; Wedell, A.; Norrby, C.; Nordenskjöld, A.; Frisén, L.; Nordenström, A. Suboptimal Psychosocial Outcomes in Patients with Congenital Adrenal Hyperplasia: Epidemiological Studies in a Nonbiased National Cohort in Sweden. *J. Clin. Endocrinol. Metab.* **2014**, *99*, 1425–1432. [CrossRef] [PubMed]
46. Faul, F.; Erdfelder, E.; Lang, A.-G.; Buchner, A. G*Power 3: A flexible statistical power analysis program for the social, behavioral, and biomedical sciences. *Behav. Res. Methods* **2007**, *39*, 175–191. [CrossRef] [PubMed]

47. Trindade, I.A.; Ferreira, C.; Pinto-Gouveia, J. The effects of body image impairment on the quality of life of non-operated Portuguese female IBD patients. *Qual. Life Res.* **2017**, *26*, 429–436. [CrossRef] [PubMed]
48. Nermoen, I.; Husebye, E.S.; Svartberg, J.; Løvås, K. Subjective health status in men and women with congenital adrenal hyperplasia: A population-based survey in Norway. *Eur. J. Endocrinol.* **2010**, *163*, 453–459. [CrossRef]
49. Bleicken, B.; Ventz, M.; Hinz, A.; Quinkler, M. Improvement of health-related quality of life in adult women with 21-hydroxylase deficiency over a seven-year period. *Endocr. J.* **2012**, *59*, 931–939. [CrossRef] [PubMed]
50. Jürgensen, M.; Kleinemeier, E.; Lux, A.; Steensma, T.D.; Cohen-Kettenis, P.T.; Hiort, O.; Thyen, U.; Köhler, B. Psychosexual Development in Adolescents and Adults with Disorders of Sex Development—Results from the German Clinical Evaluation Study. *J. Sex. Med.* **2013**, *10*, 2703–2714. [CrossRef]
51. Thyen, U.; Lux, A.; Jürgensen, M.; Hiort, O.; Köhler, B. Utilization of Health Care Services and Satisfaction with Care in Adults Affected by Disorders of Sex Development (DSD). *J. Gen. Intern. Med.* **2014**, *29*, 752–759. [CrossRef]
52. Yau, M.; Vogiatzi, M.; Lewkowitz-Shpuntoff, A.; Nimkarn, S.; Lin-Su, K. Health-Related Quality of Life in Children with Congenital Adrenal Hyperplasia. *Horm. Res. Paediatr.* **2015**, *84*, 165–171. [CrossRef]
53. Hofelmann, D.; Gonzalez-Chica, D.; Peres, K.G.; Boing, A.; Peres, M.A. Chronic diseases and socioeconomic inequalities in quality of life among Brazilian adults: Findings from a population-based study in Southern Brazil. *Eur. J. Public Heal.* **2018**, *28*, 603–610. [CrossRef] [PubMed]
54. Wu, T.-Y.; Chang, T.-W.; Chang, S.-M.; Lin, Y.-Y.; Wang, J.-D.; Kuo, Y.-L. Dynamic Changes Of Body Image And Quality Of Life In Breast Cancer Patients. *Cancer Manag. Res.* **2019**, *11*, 10563–10571. [CrossRef] [PubMed]
55. Vieira, P.N.; Palmeira, A.L.; Mata, J.; Kolotkin, R.L.; Silva, M.N.; Sardinha, L.B.; Teixeira, P.J. Usefulness of Standard BMI Cut-Offs for Quality of Life and Psychological Well-Being in Women. *Obes. Facts* **2012**, *5*, 795–805. [CrossRef] [PubMed]
56. Auer, M.K.; Ebert, T.; Pietzner, M.; Defreyne, J.; Fuss, J.; Stalla, G.K.; T'Sjoen, G. Effects of Sex Hormone Treatment on the Metabolic Syndrome in Transgender Individuals: Focus on Metabolic Cytokines. *J. Clin. Endocrinol. Metab.* **2018**, *103*, 790–802. [CrossRef]
57. Wedell, A. Molecular Genetics of 21- Hydroxylase Deficiency. *Endocr. Dev.* **2011**, *20*, 80–87. [CrossRef] [PubMed]
58. Dörr, H.-G. Adrenogenitales syndrom (AGS). In *Praktische Endokrinologie (Zweite Ausgabe)*; Allolio, B., Schulte, H.M., Eds.; Urban & Fischer: Munich, Germany, 2010; pp. 246–263.
59. Wang, L.C.; Poppas, D.P. Surgical outcomes and complications of reconstructive surgery in the female congenital adrenal hyperplasia patient: What every endocrinologist should know. *J. Steroid Biochem. Mol. Biol.* **2017**, *165*, 137–144. [CrossRef] [PubMed]
60. Hopwood, P.; Fletcher, I.; Lee, A.; Al Ghazal, S. A body image scale for use with cancer patients. *Eur. J. Cancer* **2001**, *37*, 189–197. [CrossRef]
61. Wilson, R.E.; Latner, J.D.; Hayashi, K. More than just body weight: The role of body image in psychological and physical functioning. *Body Image* **2013**, *10*, 644–647. [CrossRef]

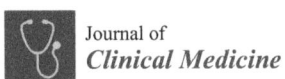

Article

Long-Term Results of Surgical Treatment and Patient-Reported Outcomes in Congenital Adrenal Hyperplasia—A Multicenter European Registry Study

Susanne Krege [1,*], Henrik Falhammar [2,3], Hildegard Lax [4], Robert Roehle [5,6], Hedi Claahsen-van der Grinten [7], Barbara Kortmann [8], Lise Duranteau [9] and Agneta Nordenskjöld [10,11] on behalf of the dsd-LIFE group

1. Department of Urology, Pediatric Urology and Urooncology, Kliniken Essen Mitte, 45136 Essen, Germany
2. Department of Endocrinology, Karolinska University Hospital, 171 77 Stockholm, Sweden
3. Department of Molecular Medicine and Surgery, Karolinska Institutet, 171 76 Stockholm, Sweden
4. Institute of Medical Informatics, Biometry and Epidemiology, University of Essen, 45147 Essen, Germany
5. Institute of Biometry and Clinical Epidemiology, Charite-University Medicine Berlin, 10117 Berlin, Germany
6. Institute of Health, Charite-University Medicine Berlin, 10117 Berlin, Germany
7. Department of Pediatric Endocrinology, Radboud University Medical Center, 6525 GA Nijmegen, The Netherlands
8. Department of Pediatric Urology, Radboud University Medical Center, 6525 GA Nijmegen, The Netherlands
9. Department of Medical Gynaecology and Reference Centre for Rare Diseases of Genital Development, Bicetre Hospital, APHP Paris Saclay University, 94270 Le Kremlin Bicetre, France
10. Department of Women's and Children's Health, Center of Molecular Medicine, Karolinska Institutet, 17176 Stockholm, Sweden
11. Department of Pediatric Surgery, Astrid Lindgren Children's Hospital, Karolinska University Hospital, 17176 Stockholm, Sweden
* Correspondence: s.krege@kem-med.com; Tel.: +49-201-174-29003; Fax: +49-201-174-29000

Abstract: Representatives for congenital adrenal hyperplasia (CAH) continue to desire early feminizing surgery in girls with 46,XX-CAH. The aim of this analysis, which included 174 46,XX- individuals with salt-wasting (SW) or simple-virilizing (SV) CAH, a female gender identity, and an age > 16 years participating in a multicenter cross-sectional clinical evaluation study (dsd-LIFE), was to evaluate the long-term results of surgery and patient-reported outcomes (PRO). The gynecological examination (n = 84) revealed some shortcomings concerning surgical feminization. A clitoris was absent in 9.5% of cases, while a clitoral hood was missing in 36.7% of cases. Though all women had large labia, they didn't look normal in 22.6% of cases. Small labia were absent in 23.8% of cases. There was no introitus vaginae, and the urethra and vagina had no separate opening in 5.1% of cases. A mucosal lining was missing in 15.4% of cases. Furthermore, 86.2% of the women had scars at the region of their external genitalia. A vaginal stenosis was described in 16.5% of cases, and a meatal stenosis was described in 2.6% of cases. Additionally, PRO data showed a very-/high satisfaction rate of 21.3%/40.2% with cosmesis and 23.8%/38.1% with functionality, while 3.3%/10.7% showed a very-/low satisfaction with cosmesis as well as 5.6%/10.3% with functionality. The remaining women—24.6% and 23.8%— were indifferent. Satisfaction concerning sex life was very-/high in 9.6%/27.7%. In 12.0%/16.9% it was very-/low. Furthermore, 33.7% had no opinion. Furthermore, 27.0%/31.6% of the women reported that clitoriplasty, but not clitoridectomy, had a very-/positive influence on their lives, while 1.3%/8.9% felt it to be very-/negative, and 28.4% were indifferent. Vaginoplasty had a very-/positive influence in 25.7%/33.8% and a very-/negative effect in 3.6%/6.8%. 29.7% had no opinion. Additionally, 75.7% of the women preferred feminizing surgery during infancy/childhood, especially concerning clitoreduction. In conclusion, though the majority of the participants (76%) preferred early feminizing surgery and 60% described a positive effect on their lives, about 10% felt it to have been negative. About 15% of the women suffered from insufficient cosmesis and functionality after surgery. Sex life was even described as poor in nearly 30%. Therefore, the decision about early genital surgery in 46,XX-CAH girls should be considered carefully. Parents should get detailed information about possible complications of surgery and should receive support to understand that postponing

Citation: Krege, S.; Falhammar, H.; Lax, H.; Roehle, R.; Claahsen-van der Grinten, H.; Kortmann, B.; Duranteau, L.; Nordenskjöld, A. Long-Term Results of Surgical Treatment and Patient-Reported Outcomes in Congenital Adrenal Hyperplasia—A Multicenter European Registry Study. *J. Clin. Med.* **2022**, *11*, 4629. https://doi.org/10.3390/jcm11154629

Academic Editor: K. Katharina Rall

Received: 27 June 2022
Accepted: 3 August 2022
Published: 8 August 2022

Publisher's Note: MDPI stays neutral with regard to jurisdictional claims in published maps and institutional affiliations.

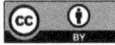

Copyright: © 2022 by the authors. Licensee MDPI, Basel, Switzerland. This article is an open access article distributed under the terms and conditions of the Creative Commons Attribution (CC BY) license (https:// creativecommons.org/licenses/by/ 4.0/).

surgery does not inevitably cause harm for their child. Importantly, genital surgery when performed in children should only be performed in expert centers with a specialized team including surgeons who are trained in feminizing surgery.

Keywords: 46,XX-DSD; congenital adrenal hyperplasia; surgical interventions; timing of surgery; patient-reported outcomes

1. Introduction

Congenital adrenal hyperplasia (CAH) is caused by adrenal enzyme defects. Its most common variant, 21-hydroxylase deficiency (21OHD), leads to deficient production of cortisol and, most often, also aldosterone, together with increased steroid precursors and androgens [1]. As a consequence, girls with classic CAH have variably virilized external genitalia at birth, with salt-wasting (SW), if there is a cortisol and aldosterone deficiency, or simply-virilized (SV), where the aldosterone production is not affected. Due to the Chicago classification from 2006, CAH belongs to the differences of sex development (DSD) [2,3]. In most Western countries, early genital surgery with the aim of achieving unambiguous female or male external genitalia in children with DSD was performed for many decades. Virilized girls with 46,XX-CAH have been surgically adapted in female direction. Depending on the severity of virilization, characterized by the Prader classification [4], this included clitoral reduction surgery—in earlier years, clitoris amputation was also performed—as well as the removal of the common urethral and vaginal duct, the so-called urogenital sinus, and the reconstruction of the distal vagina [5].

The parental concerns that atypical genitalia could have an impact on gender identity during infancy might lead parents to endorse early genital surgery. Arguments against surgery are physical damage, caused by poor cosmetic and functional results, and that is partially irreversible, as well as psychological damage in children, who are not able to decide by themselves in favor of surgery [6]. Larger series with regard to these points are hardly available. Therefore, the aim of this European multicenter registry study was to investigate the long-term outcome of genital surgery and the patient-reported outcome concerning satisfaction in women with 46,XX-CAH.

2. Methods

2.1. Study Design and Participants

This was a multicenter cross-sectional clinical evaluation study (dsd-LIFE), funded by the European Union, to evaluate the clinical care of people with DSD. The study is described in detail elsewhere [7] but is summarized below. The dsd-LIFE consortium consisted of 16 European tertiary centers from Germany, France, the Netherlands, Poland, Sweden, and the United Kingdom (UK), of which 14 were active recruiting sites. Recruitment of persons ($\geq$16 years) with DSD took place during 2014 and 2015. In total, 3100 eligible persons were approached, of whom 1040 agreed to take part in the study. All included people had a DSD condition as described in the classification system of the Chicago Consensus Conference [2,3]. All participants gave written informed consent, and the study was approved by each local ethical committee.

This study had two parts. The first included a retrospective chart review collecting data on age, class of CAH and grade of virilization at diagnosis, and time and type of surgical treatments, as well as a medical interview, with an optional gynecological/urological examination. All tasks were carried out by trained researchers, following standard operation procedures.

In the second part of the study a questionnaire about patient-reported outcomes (PRO) was analyzed.

2.2. Outcome Measurements for the Current Study

Standardized genital examination included the evaluation of external genital appearance, such as the size of clitoris or presence/absence of small labia, and functional parameters, such as the depth and width of the vagina. The examination was performed by gynecologists or urologists. Additionally, PRO related to the influence of different kinds of surgery, such as a clitoreduction/clitoridectomy and vaginoplasty, as well as vaginal dilatation, on patients' lives on a 5-point Likert scale from very negative to very positive. Another group of questions concerned genital and sexual satisfaction. Genital satisfaction was assessed by detailed evaluation of the external genitals and answering the following self-constructed questions: "Are you satisfied with the appearance of your genitals after surgery?", and "Are you satisfied with how your genitals function after surgery?" With regard to sexual satisfaction, participants were surveyed on their satisfaction with general arousability and orgasmic capacity. Lastly, participants rated their satisfaction with their sex life in general. All questions about satisfaction were rated on a 5-point Likert scale, from very dissatisfied to very satisfied. Regarding the attitudes towards surgery, participants were asked to what extent they agreed that clitoreduction is necessary in girls, if a vaginoplasty in adolescence or adulthood with a patient's consent is better than before 6 months of age, and what the preferred age for genital surgery in CAH should be (infancy/childhood, or adolescence/adulthood).

2.3. Statistical Analyses

Background, surgical data, gynecological examination, and PRO data were displayed as absolute and relative frequencies and mean ± SD or median (range) as appropriate. All proportions were calculated discounting missing values. All analyses were performed using SPSS statistics 22.0.

3. Results

In total, 226 persons with 46,XX-CAH (221 with female and 5 with male gender identity) were recruited from several European countries. Of those 221 females, 109 (49.3%) had SW-CAH, 65 (29.4%) had SV-CAH, 33 (14.9%) had NC-CAH, and 14 (6.4%) had a rare form of CAH. Of the five individuals living as males, two had SW-CAH, one SV-CAH, one NC-CAH, and one a rare form of CAH. All of these five persons, except the one with NC-CAH, underwent some kind of genital surgery/Two persons definitively had masculinization surgery, and one was operated early with feminization surgery. The analysis below only considered the 174 girls with SW- and SV-CAH, because in these subgroups feminizing surgery wasmost often performed. At birth, 8/174 (4.6%) girls had clearly female external genitals and 155/174 (89.1%) had ambiguous external genitals. In 11 cases, this information was not mentioned within the charts. Prader classification stages were reported in 112 cases. Based on clinical report forms and patient-reported data, 140/155 girls (93%) underwent operational adjustments in the female direction. Age at first surgery was available in 106 patients. Table 1 shows these basic data for the SW- and SV-CAH girls.

Table 2 shows the distribution of the different surgical procedures per CAH class. The highest percentage of both clitoris surgery and vaginoplasty was seen in the SW-CAH group. Data on the type of vaginoplasty were available for only 73 patients. The most common of these were the use of a Fortunoff flap and pedicled or free skin ($n = 55, 75.3\%$). Other procedures performed were labiaplasties ($n = 53$) and perineal plastic surgeries ($n = 32$). A vaginal dilatation was reported in 50 patients, though unfortunately data were missing in the majority of the patients.

Table 1. Basic data of 174 girls with 46,XX-CAH, subdivided into SW- and SV-CAH.

	1a: Prevalence of Prader grade by CAH class					
	Class	SW			SV	
	n	n	(%)		n	(%)
Prader grade	174	109	(62.6)		65	(37.4)
I	3	1	(33.3)		2	(66.7)
II	17	5	(29.4)		12	(70.6)
III	33	18	(54.5)		15	(45.5)
IV	50	42	(84.0)		8	(16.0)
V	9	9	(100.0)		0	
Unknown	62	34	(54.8)		28	(45.2)
	1b: Proportion of genital surgery per CAH class					
	Class	SW			SV	
	n	n	(%)		n	(%)
Surgery	174	109	(62.6)		65	(37.4)
Yes	140	89	(63.6)		51	(36.4)
	1c: Distribution of one-/two-stage genital surgery per CAH class					
	Class	SW			SV	
	n	n	(%)		n	(%)
I/II-stageOP	174	109	(62.6)		65	(37.4)
One stage	71	42	(59.2)		29	(40.8)
Two stage	48	35	(72.9)		13	(27.1)
Unknown	55	32	(58.2)		23	(41.8)
	1d: Age at first genital surgery per CAH class					
	Class	SW			SV	
	n	n	(%)		n	(%)
Age at 1. OP	174	109	(62.6)		65	(37.4)
$\leq$ 1 year	57	41	(71.9)		16	(28.1)
2–5 years	34	21	(61.8)		13	(38.2)
6–12 years	7	2	(28.6)		5	(71.4)
13–29 years	8	6	(75.0)		2	(25.0)
Unknown	68	39	(57.3)		29	(42.7)

Table 2. Proportion of surgeries per CAH class.

	Class	SW		SV	
	n	n	(%)	n	(%)
Surgery		109	(62.6)	65	(37.4)
Clitoridectomy	10	6	(60.0)	4	(40.0)
Clitoreduction	112	80	(71.4)	32	(28.6)
Vaginoplasty	121	86	(71.1)	35	(28.9)

3.1. Gynecological Examination

A gynecological examination was performed in 84 women. Median age was 28 years. A clitoris was present in 76 cases, while a clitoral hood was found in only 50 cases of them, and it was hypertrophied in 10 of these cases. Normal looking large labia were present in 65 women, while in another 19 women they rather reminded researchers of a scrotum or looked baggy. Small labia were present in 64 women, while in 20 cases no small labia could be seen. In 14 cases, an asymmetry was described. All details are given in Table 3.

Table 3. Results of the gynecological examination in 84 women with 46,XX-CAH.

Parameter	N	Yes	(%)	No	(%)
Clitoris	84	76	(90.5)	8	(9.5)
Clitoris hood	79	50	(63.3)	29	(36.7)
Large labia	84	84	(100.0)		
Small labia	84	64	(76.2)	20	(23.8)
Introitus vaginae	78	74	(94.9)	4	(5.1)
Mucosal lining	78	66	(84.6)	12	(15.4)
Separate opening for urethra and vagina	78	74	(94.9)	4	(5.1)
Vaginal length *	64	64			
Vaginal width **	73	73			
Vaginal stenosis	79	13	(16.5)	66	(83.5)
Urethrovaginal fistula	77			77	(100.0)
Meatal stenosis	77	2	(2.6)	75	(97.4)
Scars ***	80	69	(86.2)	11	(13.8)

n = number of evaluable patients. * <8 cm, n = 30 (47%); 8–10 cm, n = 31 (48%); 10–12 cm, n = 3 (5%). ** <1 finger, n = 3 (4%); one finger, n = 21 (29%); two fingers, n = 49 (67%). *** minimal, n = 45 (65.5%); moderate, n = 23 (33%); severe n = 1 (1.5%).

The overall cosmesis was rated good in 44 cases (54%), satisfactory in 35 cases (43%), and poor in 3 cases (3%) by the physician.

3.2. Patient-Reported Outcomes

Women were also surveyed about surgeries. Median age when answering the questionnaire was 28 years (range 15–64). Data differed considerably compared with the data from patients' charts. While medical charts documented clitoris surgery in 122 persons and vaginoplasty in 121, women themselves reported clitoris surgery in 88 cases, 81 in the form of a clitoris reduction, and 7 as clitoridectomy. Vaginoplasty was reported by 90 females, and 52 women mentioned that they had undergone vaginal dilatation between the age of 9 to 15 years. Information about the specified number of surgical interventions could be given by 114 women The majority had one (40%) or two (34%) surgeries, while 15% underwent three procedures, and 10.5% had more than three operations. However, the information provided does not clearly indicate the nature of subsequent interventions.

Furthermore, 99 out of 174 women (52.9%) reported to have had complications, though in 40 of them no detailed information about the kind of complication was available. Eleven women had more than one complication. Table 4 shows the rate of the most common complications. The highest rate for every complication was reported in SW-CAH.

Table 4. Overview of the most common complications according to CAH-classes.

	Class	SW		SV	
	n	n	(%)	n	(%)
Complication		109	(62.6)	65	(37.4)
Vaginal stricture	21	14	(66.7)	7	(33.3)
Scars	18	13	(72.2)	5	(27.8)
Urogenital infection	13	8	(61.5)	5	(38.5)
Urine dribbling	7	6	(85.7)	1	(14.3)

n = number of reported complications.

Table 5 shows how surgeries and vaginal dilatation influenced the women's lives. No woman mentioned clitoridectomy to have had a positive influence on her life, while nearly 60% confirmed this for clitoreduction. However, 10% denied this. The same rate of consent, respectively, denial, was reported about vaginoplasty. Concerning vaginal dilatation, 53% of the women said that it had a positive influence on their lives. Only about 11% denied this.

Table 5. Influence of surgeries and vaginal dilatation on the lives of women with 46,XX-CAH.

		Very Neg		Neg		Indifferent		Pos		Very Pos	
Procedure	n	n	(%)	n	(%)	n	(%)	n	(%)	n	(%)
Clitorireduction	74	1	(1.3)	7	(8.9)	21	(28.4)	25	(31.6)	20	(27.0)
Clitoridectomy	7	3	(42.9)	3	(42.9)	1	(14.3)	0		0	
Vaginoplasty	74	3	(3.6)	5	(6.8)	22	(29.7)	25	(33.8)	19	(25.7)
Vaginal dilatation	47	0		5	(10.6)	17	(33.3)	13	(27.7)	12	(25.5)

n = number of evaluable patients.

Table 6 summarizes the answers regarding women's satisfaction with their genitals. A very high or high satisfaction rate was reported concerning cosmesis with 61.5% satisfaction and functionality with 61.9% satisfaction, while 14% and 15.9% of the patients were very unsatisfied or unsatisfied with cosmesis and functionality. Satisfaction concerning sex life was very high or high in 37.3% of the patients, very low or low in 28.9%, and 33.7% of the patients had no opinion.

Table 6. Satisfaction with their genitals in women with 46,XX-CAH.

		Very Low		Low		Indifferent		High		Very High	
Parameter	n	n	(%)	n	(%)	n	(%)	n	(%)	n	(%)
Clitoris size	137	11	(8.0)	9	(6.6)	46	(33.6)	55	(40.1)	16	(11.7)
Clitoris shape	134	13	(9.7)	3	(2.2)	43	(32.1)	57	(42.5)	18	(13.4)
Sexual arousal	140	4	(2.9)	15	(10.7)	33	(23.6)	62	(44.3)	26	(18.6)
Orgasm	139	16	(11.5)	19	(13.7)	34	(24.5)	54	(38.8)	16	(11.5)
Vaginal length	140	0		0		46	(32.9)	73	(52.1)	21	(15.0)
Vaginal width	142	7	(4.9)	9	(6.3)	42	(29.6)	67	(47.2)	17	(12.0)
Vaginal moisture	142	5	(3.5)	28	(19.7)	40	(28.2)	58	(40.8)	11	(7.7)
Functionality	126	7	(5.6)	11	(10.3)	30	(23.8)	48	(38.1)	30	(23.8)
Cosmesis	122	4	(3.3)	13	(10.7)	30	(24.6)	49	(40.2)	26	(21.3)
Sex life	166	20	(12.0)	28	(16.9)	56	(33.7)	46	(27.7)	16	(9.6)

n = number of evaluable patients.

Additionally, three questions were related to patients' opinion on the need and timing of feminizing surgery in general. Overall, participants were questioned whether they thought that clitoral reduction surgery is necessary in girls, whether vaginoplasty in adolescence or adulthood with patient's consent is better than before 6 months of age, and about the appropriate time for genital surgery in general (Table 7). Participants were asked regardless of whether they themselves had had surgery.

Table 7. Questions concerning need and timing of feminizing surgery in women with 46,XX-CAH.

Question	n	Agree ++		Agree +		Indifferent		Disagree −		Disagree −	
		n	(%)	n	(%)	n	(%)	n	(%)	n	(%)
Need for clitoral reduction in girls	133	64	(48.1)	28	(21.0)	30	(22.6)	4	(3.0)	7	(5.3)
Vaginoplasty with patients' consent better than before 6 months	122	25	(20.5)	18	(14.7)	19	(15.6)	22	(18.0)	38	(31.1)
		Infancy		Childhood		Indifferent		Adolescence		Adulthood	
		n	(%)	n	(%)	n	(%)	n	(%)	n	(%)
Appropriate time for genital surgery	144	76	(52.8)	33	(22.9)	21	(14.6)	8	(5.6)	6	(4.2)

n = number of evaluable patients.

4. Discussion

Early genital surgery in DSD has been the subject of debate for many years. Not only do medical outcome parameters play a major role in this, but human rights issues are also a concern. Finally, the discussion has led to many countries, including Germany, to put a general ban on genital surgery for young children with DSD. However, CAH organizations do not agree with such a general ban, because they believe that the gender identity of a girl with CAH generally does not change over time and, therefore, early surgery is justified to prevent harm due to delayed surgery. The majority of persons with 46,XX- CAH identify themselves as female, and continue to prefer early feminizing surgery [8–10]. On the other hand there are reports about severely virilized 46,XX-CAH newborns assigned as males during childhood with a stable male identity in adulthood [11]. The aim of this study was to reevaluate these points, specifically surgical outcome, satisfaction rates with cosmesis and function of the genitals, and timing of surgical procedures, within a larger cohort of women with 46,XX-CAH.

Current surgical genital procedures in CAH include a modification of the clitoris, an introitoplasty and, in cases of a urogenital sinus, lifting of the sinus with reconstruction of the distal vagina. Historical descriptions about clitoral surgery favored clitoridectomy, which remained common and persisted even into the early 1980s [12]. Goodwin described the clitoris reduction with preservation of the glans and neurovascular bundle [13]. This technique underwent further refinements [14,15] and is currently the gold standard. The type of vaginoplasty depends on the Prader stage [4]. While a cut back procedure is sufficient in Prader stage I-II, higher stages require more challenging surgery. A common technique is the Fortunoff flap vaginoplasty combined with the pull-through technique depending on the length of the sinus urogenitalis [16,17]. The development of surgical techniques, especially with the intention to abandon clitoridectomy, suggest a better outcome of surgery nowadays. However, small series reporting long-term results about cosmesis and functionality after feminization do not really reflect this. Creighton et al. published long-term results of 44 adult women who underwent surgery in the early 1980s, of which 41% had a poor cosmetic result. Reintervention, mostly because of introitus or intravaginal stenosis, was necessary in 23 of 26 (89%) patients who received vaginoplasty [18]. Insufficient functionality was described by Crouch et al. and Minto et al. All patients with clitoral surgery had decreased thermal and vibratory sensitivity compared to patients without surgery and controls. All participants also received a sexual function questionnaire, which showed that patients with surgery had a lower frequency of intercourse, vaginal penetration difficulties, and a higher rate of anorgasmia [19,20]. Sircili et al. presented long-term data from 34 patients, who underwent single-stage clitorovaginoplasty between 1986 and 2002. The neurovascular bundle was preserved in only seven cases. In the other 27 patients, blood supply was only maintained by the ventral mucosa. At examination, a clitoris was visible in all 7 patients with preservation of the neurovascular bundle, but only in 21 of the other patients. Persistence of the urogenital sinus was found in 11 patients. Functional results considering menstrual flow, appearance of the introitus, and possibility of sexual intercourse were judged as excellent in 67%, good in 25%, and regular in 8% of patients [21]. Van der Zwan et al. reported about 40 patients. Of these, 36 underwent feminizing surgery, 13 as a single-stage clitorovaginoplasty at a median age of 3 years. Seven of them (54%) needed resurgery. Twenty patients underwent a two-stage procedure, clitoriplasty in early childhood, and vaginoplasty at a median age of 13. In this group, several patients needed additional surgery. In summary, 25 of the 36 patients (69%) underwent redo-operations [22].

Concerning the time for surgery, the majority of physicians preferred one-stage surgery in early childhood. Arguments from the medical side are that the tissue still possesses high elasticity in the first 3–6 months of life due to the continuing influence of the maternal estrogens, as well as the use of excess skin in clitoral reduction surgery for vaginal plastic surgery [23–28]. From a psychological point of view, the clarity of the child's genitals provides relief for parents [29]. A smaller group of surgeons favored a two-stage procedure, whereby only clitoris reduction is carried out in early childhood and a vaginoplasty is performed only at the beginning of puberty. Reasons for this are lack of indication of a vaginal reconstruction before menarche, risk of vaginal constriction caused by inadequate stretching/dilatation after early vaginal reconstruction, and long-term risk of vaginal stenosis [30–33]. If the vaginoplasty takes place only at the beginning of puberty, the girls can be trained in dilatation performed by themselves. Finally, it should be mentioned that the decision of clitoreduction within the first 6 months of life does not take into account the often remarkable effect of clitoris reduction during medical treatment.

In our study, 140/155 (93%) of the females with ambiguous genitalia underwent genital surgery. Most commonly, the time for surgery was the first year of life (57/106; 53%) or within the first 4 years (34/106; 32%). In total, 71/119 (60%) underwent a one-stage procedure, while 48/119 (40%) had a two-stage procedure. In our study, 8.5% of the girls with clitoral surgery underwent a clitoridectomy. Although the gynecological examination revealed some shortcomings, the evaluation of the surgical results by the physicians was positive in 97% of cases. However, 14% of the women were (very) unsatisfied with the cosmesis (17/122) and functionality (18/126). Sex life in general was described as (very) satisfying by only 37% (62/166) of the women. This shows that there are discrepancies between physicians and affected persons themselves when it comes to judging the surgical results, and it underlines the necessity of patient-reported outcomes, because their subjective opinion is the most important. However, the satisfaction rates may also highlight an earlier lack of information about the physical condition at birth, since females compare themselves with healthy women.

In general, surgery and even vaginal dilatation had a positive influence in about 60% of the women, except in those with clitoridectomy, which was evaluated negatively in 86% of cases. Vaginal dilatation was performed by the young women themselves between the ages of 9 to 15 years. At this time, they can understand the advantage of dilatation and will be interested in having a functioning vagina. Concerning the right time for surgery, 76% (109/144) voted for infancy and childhood, while only 10% (14/144) preferred adolescence or adulthood. When especially asked if clitoreduction is necessary in girls, 69% (92/133) agreed, but only 35% (43/122) also voted for vaginoplasty during the first 6 months of life, while 49% (60/122) preferred the latter procedure with the patient's consent.

In conclusion, this study underlines that the surgical outcome of feminizing procedures in individuals with 46,XX CAH can be optimized. Therefore, only surgeons trained in this kind of surgery should perform these procedures. Prospective registration of surgical procedures and their outcome may improve knowledge. Counseling about feminizing surgery in individuals with 46,XX-CAH should be performed in expert centers with -an multidisciplinary team to provide informed consent, especially in cases of a decision for early surgery.

The study has drawbacks since it has a cross-sectional design, and data retrieved retrospectively from the medical files are incomplete. Moreover, there is an incongruence among those data from the medical files and what patients remember, which can be seen when comparing the number of clitoral surgeries and vaginoplasties documented in the charts and what patients report. However, this might reflect the former policy not to involve patients in their situation so that they were not informed about early surgeries they underwent and do not remember. An important advantage of the study are the data of the gynecological examination and the patient-reported outcomes, though a possible bias might be that patients were primarily recruited via clinics that seem to have good experience with surgery in DSD. The gynecological examination enables a comparison about how the physicians rated the surgical results on the one side and the patients on the other side. Finally, the patients themselves gave statements about their opinions concerning time and the kind of surgery necessary. Moreover, the absence of the evaluation between specific surgical procedures and specific centers with the gynecological outcome and PRO is a great limitation.

Author Contributions: Data curation, H.L. and R.R.; Supervision, H.F., H.C.-v.d.G., B.K., L.D. and A.N.; Visualization, B.K.; Writing—original draft, S.K. All authors have read and agreed to the published version of the manuscript.

Funding: This work was supported by the European Union Seventh Framework Programme (grant 305373 [FP7/2007-2013]) and the Deutsche Forschungsgemeinschaft (Heisenberg Professorship 325768017 to NR and Projektnummer: 314061271-TRR205 to NR). The funding sources had no role in the design of the study; collection, analysis, and interpretation of the data, writing of the report; and in the decision to submit the article for publication.

Institutional Review Board Statement: The study was conducted in accordance with the Declaration of Helsinki. Ethical approvals were obtained for performance of the study by each participating centre. The ethics committee of the coordinator, which first approved the study, was the Ethics Commission of the Charité Universitätsmedizin, reference number EA2/069/13.

Informed Consent Statement: Informed consent was obtained from all subjects involved in the study.

Data Availability Statement: The datasets generated and analysed during the current study are not publicly available because data analysis will mainly be performed by the dsd-LIFE consortium. The data presented in this study are available on reasonable request from the corresponding author.

Acknowledgments: We are grateful to the persons who participated in dsd-LIFE and to all of the study centers for their enthusiasm and dedication to contact potential participants and collect high-quality data. We especially thank the support groups in the different countries that have supported the study. For an overview of all contributors we refer to our study protocol by Roehle and colleagues (2017). We publish this paper in memoriam and with the greatest thanks to PD Birgit Köhler (Charite Universitatsmedizin, Berlin), the principle investigator of the European consortium dsd-LIFE, deceased in March 2019. We honour Birgit Köhler's dedicated leadership, energy and enthusiasm for the dsd-LIFE project and her promotion of collaboration of clinicians, patients and support groups–aiming to improve clinical care for "differences/disorders of sex development". **The dsd-LIFE Group:** Birgit Köhler and Uta Neumann, Berlin; Peggy Cohen-Kettenis, Baudewijntje Kreukels and Annelou de Vries, Amsterdam; Wiebke Arlt, Birmingham; Claudia Wiesemann, Gottingen; Jolanta Slowikowska-Hilczer, Lodz; Ute Thyen and Marion Rapp, Lubeck; Aude Brac de la Perriere, Lyon; Charles Sultan and Francoise Paris, Montpellier; Nicole Reisch, Munich; Annette Richter-Unruh, Münster and Bochum; Hedi Claahsen-van der Grinten, Nijmegen; Claire Bouvattier and Lise

Duranteau, Paris; Anna Nordenström and Agneta Nordenskjöld, Stockholm; Catherine Pienkowski, Toulouse; Maria Szarras-Czapnik, Warsaw.

Conflicts of Interest: The authors declare no conflict of interest.

References

1. Claahsen-van der Grinten, H.L.; Speiser, P.W.; Ahmed, S.F.; Arlt, W.; Auchus, R.J.; Falhammar, H.; Flück, C.E.; Guasti, L.; Huebner, A.; Kortmann, B.B.M.; et al. Congenital adrenal hyperplasia—Current insights in pathophysiology, diagnostics and management. *Endocr. Rev.* **2022**, *43*, 91–159. [CrossRef] [PubMed]
2. Hughes, I.A.; Houk, C.P.; Ahmed, S.F.; Lee, P.A.; LWPES Consensus Group; ESPE Consensus Group. Consensus statement on management of intersex disorders. *Arch. Dis. Child.* **2006**, *91*, 554–563. [CrossRef] [PubMed]
3. Lee, P.A.; Nordenström, A.; Houk, C.P.; Ahmed, S.F.; Auchus, R.; Baratz, A.; Baratz Dalke, K.; Liao, L.-M.; Lin-Su, K.; Looijenga, L.H.J.; et al. Global disorders of sex development, update since 2006: Perceptions, approach and care. *Horm. Res. Paediatr.* **2016**, *85*, 158–180. [CrossRef] [PubMed]
4. Prader, A. Genital findings in the female pseudo-hermaphroditism of the congenital adrenogenital syndrome; morphology, frequency, development and heredity of the different genital forms. *Helv. Paediatr. Acta* **1954**, *9*, 231–248. [PubMed]
5. Braga, L.H.; Salle, J.L.P. Congenital adrenal hyperplasia: A critical appraisal of the evolution of feminizing genitoplasty and the controversies surrounding gender reassignment. *Eur. J. Paediatr. Surg.* **2009**, *19*, 203–210. [CrossRef]
6. Lossie, A.C.; Green, J. Building trust: The history and ongoing relationships amongst DSD clinicians, researchers, and patient advocacy groups. *Horm. Metab. Res.* **2015**, *47*, 344–350. [CrossRef]
7. Roehle, R.; on behalf of the dsd-LIFE Group; Gehrmann, K.; Szarras-Czapnik, M.; der Grinten, H.C.-V.; Pienkowski, C.; Bouvattier, C.; Cohen-Kettenis, P.; Nordenström, A.; Thyen, U.; et al. Participation of adults with disorders/differences of sex development (DSD) in the clinical study dsd-LIFE: Design, methology, recruitment, data quality and study population. *BMC Endocr. Disord.* **2017**, *17*, 26. [CrossRef]
8. Babu, R.; Shah, U. Gender identity disorder (GID) in adolescents and adults with differences of sex development (DSD): A systematic review and meta-analysis. *J. Paediatr. Urol.* **2021**, *17*, 39–47. [CrossRef]
9. German Ethics Council. Intersexuality Opinion 2012. Available online: https://www.ethikrat.org/fileadmin/Publikationen/Stellungnahmen/englisch/opinion-intersexuality.pdf (accessed on 20 March 2022).
10. Kreukels, B.P.C.; Köhler, B.; Nordenström, A.; Roehle, R.; Thyen, U.; Bouvattier, C.; de Vries, A.L.; Cohen-Kettenis, P.T.; Arlt, W.; Wiesemann, C.; et al. Gender dysphoria and gender changes in disorders of sex development/intersex condition: Results from the dsd.LIFE Group. *J. Sex. Med.* **2018**, *15*, 777–785. [CrossRef]
11. Khattab, A.; Yau, M.; Qamar, A.; Gangishetti, P.; Barhen, A.; Al-Malki, S.; Mistry, H.; Anthony, W.; Toralles, M.; New, M.I. Long term outcomes in 46,XX adult patients with congenital adrenal hyperplasia reared as males. *J. Steroid Biochem. Mol. Biol.* **2017**, *165*, 12–17. [CrossRef]
12. Young, H.H. *Genital Abnormalities, Hermaphroditism, and Related Adrenal Diseases*; William and Wilkins: Baltimore, MD, USA, 1937; pp. 274–275.
13. Goodwin, W.E. Surgical revision of the enlarged clitoris. In *American College of Surgeons and Deutsche Gesellschaft für Chirurgie (Joint Meeting, Munich 1968)*; de la Camp, H.B., Linder, F., Trede, M., Eds.; Springer: New York, NY, USA, 1969; p. 256.
14. Kogan, S.J.; Smey, P.; Levitt, S.B. Subtunical reduction clitoroplasty: A safe modification of existing techniques. *J. Urol.* **1983**, *130*, 746–748. [CrossRef]
15. Baskin, L.S.; Erol, A.; Li, Y.W.; Liu, W.H.; Kurzrock, E.; Cunha, G.R. Anatomical studies of the human clitoris. *J. Urol.* **1999**, *162*, 1015–1020. [CrossRef]
16. Fortunoff, S.; Lattimer, J.K.; Edson, M. Vaginoplasty technique for female pseudoherma-phroditism. *Surg. Gynecol. Obstet.* **1964**, *188*, 543–548.
17. Hendren, W.H.; Crawford, J.D. Adrenogenital syndrome: The anatomy of the anomaly and its repair. Some new concepts. *J. Paediatr. Surg.* **1969**, *4*, 49–58. [CrossRef]
18. Creighton, S.M.; Minto, C.L.; Steele, S.J. Objective cosmetic and anatomical outcomes at adolescence of feminizing surgery for ambiguous genitalia done in childhood. *Lancet* **2001**, *358*, 124–125. [CrossRef]
19. Crouch, N.S.; Liao, L.M.; Woodhouse, C.R.J.; Conway, G.S.; Creighton, S.M. Sexual function and genital sensitivity following feminizing genitoplasty for congenital adrenal hyperplasia. *J. Urol.* **2008**, *179*, 634–638. [CrossRef]
20. Minto, C.L.; Liao, L.M.; Woodhouse, R.J.; Ransley, P.G.; Creighton, S.M. The effect of clitoral surgery on sexual outcome in individuals who have intersex conditions with ambiguous genitalia: A cross-sectional study. *Lancet* **2003**, *361*, 1252–1257. [CrossRef]
21. Sircili, M.H.P.; de Mendonca, B.B.; Denes, F.T.; Madureira, G.; Bachega, T.A.S.S.; Silva, F.A.D.Q.E. Anatomical and functional outcomes of feminizing genitoplasty for ambiguous genitalia in patients with virilizing congenital adrenal hyperplasia. *Clinics* **2006**, *61*, 209–214. [CrossRef]
22. Van der Zwan, Y.G.; Janssen, E.H.; Callens, N.; Wolffenbuttel, K.P.; Cohen-Kettenis, P.T.; Berg, M.V.D.; Drop, S.L.; Dessens, A.B.; Beerendonk, C. Severity of virilization is associated with cosmetic appearance and sexual function in women with congenital adrenal hyperplasia: A cross-sectional study. *J. Sex. Med.* **2013**, *10*, 866–875. [CrossRef]

23. Gonzalez, R.; Fernandes, E.T. Single stage feminization genitoplasty. *J. Urol.* **1990**, *143*, 776–778. [CrossRef]
24. Donahoe, P.K.; Gustafson, M.L. Early one-stage surgical reconstruction of the extremely high vagina in patients with congenital adrenal hyperplasia. *J. Pediatr. Surg.* **1994**, *29*, 352–358. [CrossRef]
25. De Jong, T.P.V.; Boemers, T.M.L. Neonatal management of female intersex by clitorovaginaoplasty. *J. Urol.* **1995**, *154*, 830–832. [CrossRef]
26. Rink, R.C.; Adams, M.C. Feminizing genitoplasty: State of art. *World J. Urol.* **1998**, *16*, 212–218. [CrossRef] [PubMed]
27. Farkas, A.; Chertin, B. Feminizing genitoplasty in patients with 46XX congenital adrenal hyperplasia. *J. Pediatr. Endocrionl. Metab.* **2001**, *14*, 713–722. [CrossRef] [PubMed]
28. Creighton, S.M.; Farhat, W.A. Early versus late intervention of congenital adrenal hyperplasia. *J. Pediatr. Adolesc. Gynecol.* **2005**, *18*, 63–69. [CrossRef]
29. Binet, A.; Lardy, H.; Geslin, D.; Francois-Fiquet, C.; Poli-Merol, M.L. Should we question early feminizing genitoplasty for patients with congenital adrenal hyperplasia and XX karyotype? *J. Pediatr. Surg.* **2016**, *51*, 465–468. [CrossRef]
30. Creighton, S.M. Feminizing surgery: What should be done and when? *J. Pediatr. Adolesc. Gynecol.* **2005**, *18*, 63–69. [CrossRef]
31. Creighton, S.; Chernausek, S.D.; Romao, R.; Ransley, P.; PippiSalle, J. Timing and nature of reconstructive surgery for disorders of sex development—Introduction. *J. Pediatr. Urol.* **2012**, *8*, 602–610. [CrossRef]
32. Krege, S.; Walz, K.H.; Hauffa, B.P.; Körner, I.; Rübben, H. Long-term follow-up of female patients with congenital adrenal hyperplasia from 21-hydroxylase deficiency, with special emphasis on the results of vaginoplasty. *Br. J. Urol.* **2000**, *86*, 253–259. [CrossRef]
33. Gastaud, F.; Bouvattier, C.; Duranteau, L.; Brauner, R.; Thibaud, E.; Kutten, F.; Bougnères, P. Impaired sexual and reproductive outcomes in women with classical forms of congenital adrenal hyperplasia. *J. Clin. Endocrinol. Metab.* **2007**, *92*, 1391–1396. [CrossRef]

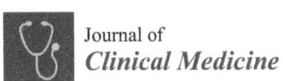

Article

MYRF: A New Regulator of Cardiac and Early Gonadal Development—Insights from Single Cell RNA Sequencing Analysis

Verónica Calonga-Solís [1,2], Helena Fabbri-Scallet [1,3], Fabian Ott [2], Mostafa Al-Sharkawi [1,4], Axel Künstner [2], Lutz Wünsch [5], Olaf Hiort [1], Hauke Busch [2] and Ralf Werner [1,6,*]

1. Division of Paediatric Endocrinology and Diabetes, Department of Paediatric and Adolescent Medicine, University of Lübeck, 23562 Lübeck, Germany
2. Medical Systems Biology Division, Lübeck Institute of Experimental Dermatology, University of Lübeck, 23562 Lübeck, Germany
3. Center for Molecular Biology and Genetic Engineering—CBMEG, State University of Campinas, Campinas 13083-875, Brazil
4. Biochemical Genetics Department, Human Genetics and Genome Research Institute, National Research Centre, Dokki, Cairo 12622, Egypt
5. Department of Pediatric Surgery, University of Lübeck, 23562 Lübeck, Germany
6. Institute of Molecular Medicine, University of Lübeck, 23562 Lübeck, Germany
* Correspondence: ralf.werner@uni-luebeck.de

Abstract: De novo variants in the myelin regulatory factor (MYRF), a transcription factor involved in the differentiation of oligodendrocytes, have been linked recently to the cardiac and urogenital syndrome, while familiar variants are associated with nanophthalmos. Here, we report for the first time on a patient with a de novo stop-gain variant in *MYRF* (p.Q838*) associated with Scimitar syndrome, 46,XY partial gonadal dysgenesis (GD) and severe hyperopia. Since variants in *MYRF* have been described in both 46,XX and 46,XY GD, we assumed a role of *MYRF* in the early development of the bipotential gonad. We used publicly available single cell sequencing data of human testis and ovary from different developmental stages and analysed them for *MYRF* expression. We identified *MYRF* expression in the subset of coelomic epithelial cells at stages of gonadal ridge development in 46,XX and 46,XY individuals. Differential gene expression analysis revealed significantly upregulated genes. Within these, we identified *CITED2* as a gene containing a MYRF binding site. It has been shown that *Cited2*$^{-/-}$ mice have gonadal defects in both testis and ovary differentiation, as well as defects in heart development and establishment of the left–right axis. This makes *MYRF* a potential candidate as an early regulator of gonadal and heart development via upregulation of the transcriptional cofactor *CITED2*.

Keywords: *MYRF*; *CITED2*; scimitar syndrome; disorders of sex development; gonadal development; cardiac and urogenital syndrome

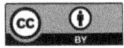

1. Introduction

In 2009, the *MYRF* gene (*Myelin Regulatory Factor*, OMIM * 608329) was described as a critical transcriptional regulator required for the myelination of the central nervous system (CNS) [1]. Subsequently, studies characterized the function of *MYRF* as a membrane-associated transcription factor for oligodendrocyte differentiation, stimulating myelin gene expression in the CNS [2,3]. Currently, it is known that *MYRF* is also expressed in other tissues in addition to the CNS, especially during the early development of the diaphragm, heart, eyes, lungs and genitourinary tract, which is consistent with the fact that variants in this gene have been associated with congenital diaphragmatic hernia [4], congenital heart diseases [5], nanophthalmos and other ocular defects [6], and more recently, with a new cardiac and urogenital syndrome (CUGS), as well as with disorders/differences of sex development (DSD) [7,8], a group of conditions in which development of chromosomal, gonadal or anatomic sex is atypical [9]. Sex determination in mammals is controlled by the interaction between many genes that drive a bistable embryonic gonadal development program. Testis and ovarian promoting pathways act as an antagonistic network system with a remarkable plasticity [10]. In the 46,XY gonad, the presence of SRY activates the *SOX9/FGF9* pathway, leading to testis development, Sertoli and Leydig cell formation and androgen production, resulting to internal and external virilization. In contrast, the absence of *SRY* in the 46,XX gonad will upregulate the *RSPO1/WNT4/b-catenin* pathway, repressing the *SOX9/FGF9* pathway to promote ovarian development, with granulosa and theca cells. In humans, a disruption in either pathway can result in gonadal dysgenesis, leading to a range of genital phenotypes between both sexes [11].

MYRF (previously known as *C11orf9* [12]), is located at 11q12.2 and expands around 35 kb of genomic DNA divided into 27 exons. It encodes for a 1151 amino acid protein, characterized by a proline-rich region containing a nuclear localization signal (NLS), a DNA-binding domain (DBD), an intramolecular chaperone auto-processed domain (ICA) (also known as Peptidase S74 domain), a transmembrane domain (TM) and two myelin gene regulatory factor C-terminal domains (MRF C1 and MRF C2) [3,12]. An intramolecular chaperone from the ICA domain helps *MYRF* to form a homo-trimer in the endoplasmic reticulum, which is essential for its biological process, where it carries out the auto-cleavage of *MYRF*, allowing it to function as a transcription factor in the nucleus [13].

Here, we report a novel, heterozygous de novo p.Q838* variant in *MYRF* in a patient with 46,XY partial gonadal dysgenesis (PGD), Scimitar syndrome and severe hyperopia, identified by whole genome analysis. Haploinsufficiency of *MYRF* has been identified as a cause of DSD in 46,XX and 46,XY individuals [7]; however, there is limited knowledge about the function of this gene and its influence on the molecular pathways in sex development. To elucidate the influence of *MYRF* expression on the developing gonads, we use previously published single cell RNA-seq data of human testes and ovaries. *CITED2* was found upregulated in *MYRF*-expressing cells and is possibly a downstream target of *MYRF*. We highlight the important role *MYRF* plays in early developmental stages of the undifferentiated gonad and how it can affect gonadal development of 46,XY and 46,XX individuals, as well as heart morphogenesis and establishment of the left–right axis.

2. Materials and Methods

2.1. Patient Description

The child was prenatally suspected of having a congenital heart defect with questionable situs inversus and anomalous pulmonary vein confluence. The birth was by caesarean section at gestational week 38 + 5. Genital status was not questioned at that time and a female sex was assigned. Scimitar syndrome was diagnosed with dextrocardia and an abnormal confluence of a right-sided pulmonary vein in the inferior vena cava. The right lung showed a rudimentary upper lobe bronchus that narrowed after 1 cm. Only one dorsal relatively small right upper lobe segment was present. The right lower lobe was pushed dorsally by the heart and was considerably compressed and partly atelectatic. Moreover, also belonging to the right lung, an overinflating lung segment was seen ventrobasally to the left of the heart. The well ventilated and fully expanded left lung was considerably larger than the right one. In addition, aside of the spleen, two small accessory spleens were seen. At the age of 6 months, the anomalous pulmonary veins became attached to the left atrium. A follow-up at the age of one year showed rarefaction in the right lower lobe of the lung.

At the age of 8 years, clitoris hypertrophy without signs of puberty became apparent and the child was seen by a paediatric endocrinologist. Apparently, both gonadotrophins and testosterone were elevated. She presented to our hospital endocrine unit at the age of 10 years for further assessment. At this time, she felt healthy and there were no imminent pulmonary or cardiovascular problems. She had no acne, no hirsutism, no breast development and was of normal height and weight. She had severe hyperopia with 9 dpt, corrected with glasses. Her clitoris was 3.5 cm in length and the labia majora were rugated. LH was 5.7 IU/L (within the adult range), FSH 69.9 IU/L (above adult range), testosterone 0.51 µg/L (elevated for the female reference range, within the reference range of Tanner 2 pubertal development for boys). Additionally, 17-beta estradiol was below detection and inhibin B, at 9 pg/mL, was below the reference range for boys. On ultrasound, she had a small tubular structure behind the bladder, which was interpreted as a small rudimentary uterus. This was confirmed by MRI; gonads could not be visualised at that time. Urine steroid metabolome analysis revealed no signs of congenital adrenal hypoplasia. Subsequent karyotype analysis was 46,XY (ishYP11.3, SRY positive). Taken together, the findings were consistent with a 46,XY PGD. Puberty was stopped by a GnRH analogue. After gender assessment by a psychologist, puberty was induced at an appropriate age by estrogens/progestins. During follow-up, small gonads could be visualized by ultrasound or MRI in the inguinal canal and were examined every 12 months. Prophylactic gonadectomy was discussed repeatedly and a shared decision was made to delay the procedure until after her 18th birthday. Dextrocardia and hyperopia in conjunction with gonadal dysgenesis suggested a syndromic form of DSD. Array-CGH using a 180 k Microarray (Agilent) revealed an unsuspicious 46,XY karyotype without clinical relevant deletions or duplications (arr [hg19] 1–22)x2,(XY)x1). To elucidate the cause of this form of DSD, a whole genome sequencing analysis was initiated.

2.2. Whole Genome Sequencing (WGS)

WGS was performed to identify putative pathogenic variants, indels and structural variations. Sequencing libraries were constructed from 1.0 µg DNA per sample using the Truseq Nano DNA HT Sample Preparation Kit (Illumina, San Diego, CA, USA), following the recommendations of the manufacturer. Genomic DNA was randomly fragmented to a size of approximately 350 bp by Covaris cracker (Covaris, Woburn, MA, USA). DNA fragments were blunted, A-tailed and ligated with the full-length adapter for Illumina sequencing with further PCR amplification. Libraries were purified using AMPure XP (Beckman Coulter, Pasadena, CA, USA), analysed for size distribution on an Agilent 2100 Bioanalyser (Agilent Technologies, Santa Clara, CA, USA) and quantified by qPCR. Paired end sequencing of libraries was performed on Illumina HiSeq platforms (Illumina). Per sample, more than 90 GB of raw data were obtained, resulting in an average genomic read depth of $30\times$.

2.3. Bioinformatics

Sequencing reads were mapped to human reference genome version GRCh38 using the Burrows–Wheeler Aligner (BWA-MEM, v0.7.17) [14], and resulting mapping files were processed following GATK (Genome Analysis Toolkit) best practices for germline variant calling. Briefly, we screened for duplicated reads by applying *Mark Duplicates* from Picard tools (v.2.26.1, http://broadinstitute.github.io/picard/, accessed on 3 September 2021); split-reads and discordant paired-end alignments were extracted using *SAM tools* v0.1.18 [14] as implemented in (GATK, v.4.2.2.0) [15] with standard parameters. Single nucleotide variants (SNVs) and short insertions/deletions (InDels) were called using *Deep Variant* (v1.2.0). Detection of structural variants (SV) was performed using DELLY [16]. Variants were annotated using Ensembl Variant Effect Predictor—VEP (v103) (EMBL-EBI, Cambridge, UK). All chromosomal positions in the paper are according to GRCh38.

2.4. Single Cell RNA Analyses

We analysed publicly available single-cell RNA from testes and ovaries, which totalled 20 samples from testes of individuals at different stages, from embryo to adult men, and 4 samples of ovaries, from embryos and foetus [17–20] (for more detail, see the *Data Availability* section below and Supplementary Table S1). The scRNA sequences of these samples were obtained through the 10x Genomics sequencing platform. We pre-processed the raw sequences using fastp (v0.22.0) [21], which were later aligned and annotated to the human reference cDNA GRCh38 with Kallisto (v0.46.1) and BUStools (v0.39.3) [22]. This resulted in matrixes of UMI counts for each sample. The downstream filtering and analyses were performed with the R package Seurat v4.1.1 [23]. In brief, we retained genes expressed in at least three cells, and we kept cells if they had less than 25% reads mapping to the mitochondrial genome, if they had between 500 and 9000 genes, and if they had less than 40,000 mRNA molecules detected. We normalized the gene counts in each cell by the total cell expression, with the *Normalize Data* function, using log10-transformation and a scale factor of 10,000. Integration of the samples was performed for testes and ovaries datasets separately, using *FindIntegration Anchors* and *Integrate Data* functions. Afterward, the cells were clustered by a shared nearest neighbour (SNN) modularity optimization and visualized in a two-dimensional space based on uniform manifold approximation and projection (UMAP). We classified the cell populations using the same marker genes as in the original publications [17–20] and other published literature [24,25].

To investigate which genes could have their expression affected by *MYRF*, we first subset the cell cluster of the coelomic epithelium (CE), the cell population that expressed this gene the highest. Later, we performed a differential expression analysis between the cells that express *MYRF* against those that do not express it, using the *FindMarkers* function with default parameters.

3. Results

We performed Trio-WGS (mother, father and affected child) and focused our analyses on protein-coding regions. SNVs and Indels were filtered for rare variants (frequency in 1 k project or gnomAD below 0.1%). A heterozygous de novo stop-gain variant in exon 20 of the myelin regulatory factor (*MYRF*) was detected (NM_001127392:c.2512C>T; p.Q838*) and confirmed by Sanger sequencing (Figure 1). According to the ACMG guidelines [26], this variant was considered pathogenic as it fulfils two criteria of the evidence of pathogenicity: PSV1 (classified as "null variant" since it is a nonsense variant) and PS1 (de novo variant confirmed by the absence in both parents). De novo variants in *MYRF* have been recently detected in patients with CUGS [27]. No further variants in genes associated with gonadal dysgenesis have been detected.

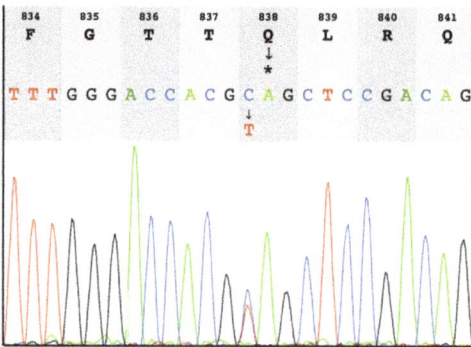

Figure 1. Sanger chromatogram showing the de novo heterozygous stop-gain variant in *MYRF* (c.2512C>T; p.Q838*) in the study patient.

Since variants in *MYRF* have been recently detected not only in 46,XY, but also 46,XX gonadal dysgenesis [7], we hypothesized that heterozygous inactivating variants may affect very early development of the bipotential gonad. Therefore, we reanalysed publicly available single cell RNA sequencing data (scRNA-seq) of different stages of human gonadal development to study the impact that *MYRF* could have in the early development of the gonads.

According to their stage or age, the testis samples were classified as embryonic, foetal, mini puberty, peri-puberty, pre-puberty and adults, and the ovary samples were classified as embryonic or foetal (Supplementary Table S1). The reanalysis of these datasets yielded ~111,000 cells from testes and ~28,000 cells from the ovaries, which clustered in 20 and 19 cell populations, respectively (Figure 2), which were identified according to their distinctive gene expression (Supplementary Figures S1 and S2). In testes, clusters 1–7 were annotated as Leydig cells, clusters 8–10 as Sertoli cells. Cluster 11 was classified as mesonephric cells; however, it was also composed of cells with gene expression patterns of Leydig and Sertoli cells and was present mainly in the embryos and foetus. Cluster 12 was identified as coelomic epithelium cells and was also present mainly in embryos and foetus. Cluster 14–15 belonged to germ cells. The remaining clusters were classified as peritubular myoid, endothelial, macrophages and blood cells (Figure 2A). In ovaries, theca cells were found in cluster 1–6, granulosa cells in cluster 7–10, mesonephric cells in cluster 11 and coelomic epithelium cells in cluster 12. Germ cells were present in cluster 14–15 and the remaining cells were classified as smooth muscle, endothelial, macrophages and blood cells (Figure 2B).

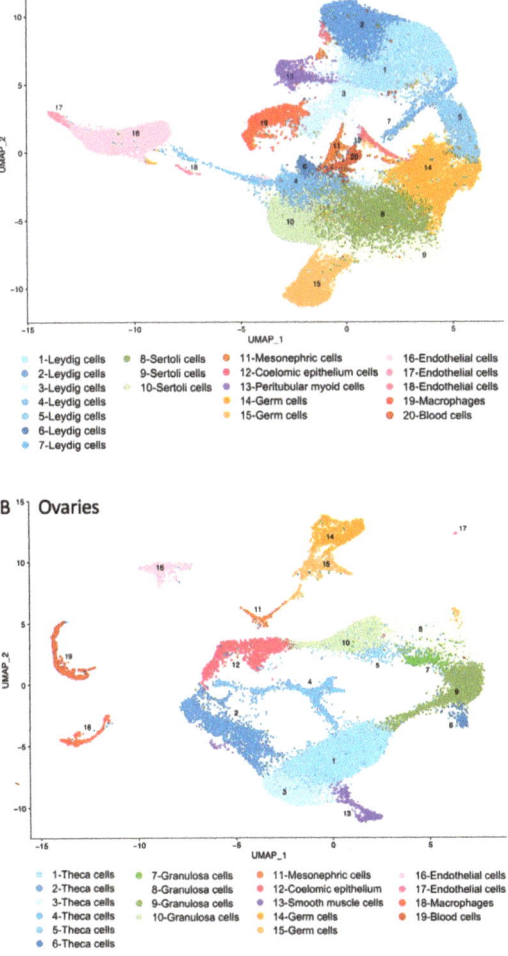

Figure 2. UMAP plots of cell clusters in human (**A**) testes from embryonic stage to adults; and (**B**) ovaries from embryonic and foetal stages identified by single cell RNA sequencing. UMAP: uniform manifold approximation and projection.

We observed that, in both testes and ovaries, *MYRF* is highly expressed in a subset of cells from the coelomic epithelium (CE) at embryonic and foetal stages (Figure 3), and that its expression is lowered after birth (Supplementary Figure S3). We aimed to search for genes that might be directly or indirectly regulated by this transcription factor. Therefore, we divided the cluster of CE cells into cells that express *MYRF* and those that do not, and investigated them for differentially expressed (DE) genes. We found 62 DE genes in the CE cells of testis and 13 genes in the CE of ovaries. Within this set of DE genes, approximal half of them (26 of the testis and 7 of the ovary genes) have *MYRF* binding sites according to the *GeneHancer* database [28] (Tables 1 and 2). One of these DE genes, the *CBP/p300-interacting transactivator with Glu/Asp-rich carboxy-terminal domain 2* (*CITED2*), is of particular interest, since it is a transcriptional cofactor that acts in the early stages of XX and XY gonadal development [29,30], and is involved in heart morphogenesis and establishment of the left–right axis [31].

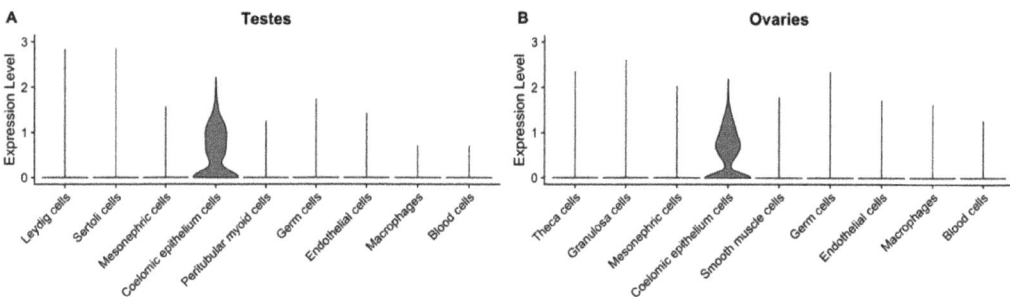

Figure 3. Expression levels of *MYRF* in testes (**A**) and ovaries (**B**) at embryonic and fetal stages, showing that it is highly expressed in coelomic epithelium cells.

Table 1. List of genes differentially expressed between the cells that express *MYRF* and those that do not, in the coelomic epithelium cluster of ovaries.

				Female Samples					
DE Genes	Binding Site for MYRF	pct. MYRF (+)	pct. MYRF (−)	*p*-Value adj	DE Genes	Binding Site for MYRF	pct. MYRF (+)	pct. MYRF (−)	*p*-Value adj
MYRF	+	1	0	1.3608×10^{-261}	ZFP36	+	0.543	0.398	3.03465×10^{-5}
NR4A1	−	0.444	0.249	1.63171×10^{-10}	IER2	+	0.81	0.691	0.000188878
SOCS3	−	0.443	0.239	2.54304×10^{-10}	CITED2	+	0.672	0.474	0.000278465
CRIP1	−	0.509	0.322	5.59507×10^{-8}	CALB2	−	0.439	0.292	0.000329296
FOSB	+	0.568	0.383	1.88434×10^{-7}	JUNB	+	0.642	0.513	0.001629543
EGR1	+	0.631	0.464	1.82088×10^{-6}	FOS	−	0.775	0.693	0.006444703
DUSP1	+	0.644	0.459	3.9062×10^{-6}					

DE: differential expression analyses. *MYRF* (+): cells from coelomic epithelium that express at least one transcript of *MYRF*. *MYRF* (−): cells from coelomic epithelium that do not express any transcript of *MYRF*. Pct: percentage of cells where the gene is detected in *MYRF* (+) or (−) subsets.

Table 2. List of genes differentially expressed between the cells that express *MYRF* and those that do not, in the coelomic epithelium cluster of testes.

				Male Samples					
DE Genes	Binding Site for MYRF	pct. MYRF (+)	pct. MYRF (−)	*p*-Value adj	DE Genes	Binding Site for MYRF	pct. MYRF (+)	pct. MYRF (−)	*p*-Value adj
MYRF	+	1	0	1.18×10^{-81}	TNNI1	−	0.764	0.45	0.001116
H2AFX	+	0.651	0.282	6.08×10^{-8}	TMEM88	−	0.455	0.187	0.001454
C21orf58	−	0.371	0.1	1.29×10^{-6}	GGH	−	0.48	0.201	0.001921
HILPDA	−	0.535	0.201	2.98×10^{-6}	UBE2T	−	0.455	0.211	0.001941
DSG2	+	0.549	0.211	3.24×10^{-6}	MKI67	−	0.404	0.163	0.002216
DNMT1	+	0.6	0.263	3.39×10^{-6}	ZWINT	−	0.484	0.22	0.002686

Table 2. Cont.

				Male Samples					
DE Genes	Binding Site for MYRF	pct. MYRF (+)	pct. MYRF (−)	p-Value adj	DE Genes	Binding Site for MYRF	pct. MYRF (+)	pct. MYRF (−)	p-Value adj
ROBO1	−	0.484	0.172	8.73×10^{-6}	CDK1	−	0.418	0.172	0.002747
AURKB	+	0.458	0.163	2.32×10^{-5}	IDH2	+	0.698	0.407	0.003044
SGO1	−	0.371	0.11	3.15×10^{-5}	CDCA3	−	0.313	0.1	0.004612
GMNN	+	0.524	0.225	3.97×10^{-5}	PABPN1	+	0.76	0.488	0.004802
NOVA1	−	0.716	0.383	4.61×10^{-5}	MTRNR2L10	NA	0.825	0.526	0.006358
STX10	+	0.585	0.258	7.52×10^{-5}	PCNA	+	0.665	0.373	0.006529
UBE2S	+	0.625	0.335	9.06×10^{-5}	TYRO3	+	0.633	0.325	0.008898
CMSS1	−	0.622	0.297	0.000107	ECI1	+	0.596	0.306	0.009338
FEN1	−	0.447	0.172	0.000119	TK1	+	0.564	0.325	0.009615
SCARB2	+	0.629	0.306	0.000145	EIF3E	+	0.982	0.967	0.010135
RPSAP52	−	0.444	0.172	0.000187	LAPTM4B	−	0.895	0.67	0.011395
HNRNPAB	+	0.716	0.388	0.000202	CKS2	+	0.695	0.426	0.014009
YLPM1	−	0.407	0.148	0.000275	RABL6	−	0.651	0.368	0.01407
LIG1	+	0.349	0.11	0.000322	CENPF	−	0.524	0.282	0.015355
SMC1A	−	0.455	0.182	0.000419	AKR1B1	+	0.876	0.617	0.020538
SMC2	−	0.498	0.225	0.000429	BIRC5	+	0.545	0.311	0.021154
H2AFZ	−	0.942	0.823	0.00049	AURKA	+	0.255	0.077	0.021308
CENPM	−	0.44	0.177	0.000496	CBX5	+	0.931	0.732	0.022631
CENPV	−	0.647	0.368	0.000586	SMARCC1	+	0.771	0.464	0.022672
USP10	−	0.531	0.244	0.000751	UBE2C	+	0.542	0.297	0.023105
CDH3	−	0.531	0.249	0.000837	ZDHHC8P1	−	0.742	0.464	0.027005
ASF1B	+	0.302	0.086	0.000849	MAG	−	0.495	0.249	0.031231
HNRNPD	+	0.884	0.718	0.00087	SOX11	−	0.64	0.383	0.031795
ITGA3	−	0.596	0.292	0.000892	TPX2	+	0.375	0.153	0.035526
TMEM106C	−	0.68	0.411	0.000936	H2AFV	−	0.858	0.622	0.038892
FBXO5	−	0.367	0.129	0.000963					

DE: differential expression analyses. MYRF (+): cells from coelomic epithelium that express at least one transcript of MYRF. MYRF (−): cells from coelomic epithelium that do not express any transcript of MYRF. Pct: percentage of cells where the gene is detected in MYRF (+) or (−) subsets.

4. Discussion

The MYRF gene encodes a membrane-associated transcription factor, which has been recently identified as candidate of a new syndrome of cardiac and urogenital anomalies (CUGS) [27,32]. Shortly afterwards, further de novo variants in MYRF have been identified as the genetic cause of congenital diaphragmatic hernia (CDH) in patients that also presented congenital heart disease (CHD); three of the patients also had varying genital anomalies ranging from female external genitalia with a blind ending vagina to ambiguous genitalia and/or undescended testes, extending the spectrum of CUGS [4].

Additionally, variants in MYRF have been found in patients with eye conditions. For instance, Garnai and colleagues [6] identified a frameshift variant (c.769dupC, p.S264Qfs*74) in an eight year old male subject with nanophtahalmos, an extreme form of hyperopia or farsightedness, who presented cardiac and urogenital malformations, such as a mitral valve prolapse, a micropenis and unilateral cryptorchidism. In the same way, Xiao and colleagues [33] found a de novo frameshift variant (c.3274_3275del, p.L1093Pfs*22) in a six year old boy with high hyperopia and a splice-site variant (c.3194 + 2T>C) in a 40-year-old woman with high hyperopia that developed angle-closure glaucoma of both eyes. Familial cases of nanophthalmos due to disrupting variants of MYRF have also been identified. Garnai and colleagues also studied a large family with inherited nanophthalmos, and found a disrupting splice site variant (c.3376-1G>A, p.G1126Vfs*31), leading to a frameshift in the last exon. Four members of this family also had dextrocardia, and one of them also had a right hypoplastic lung and pulmonary artery stenosis. Shortly after, Xiao and colleagues [33], investigating another large family with inherited nanophthalmos, revealed an additional truncating mutation in MYRF (c.3377delG, p.G1126Vfs*31). Although the variants in the two large families identified by Garnai et al. [6] and Xiao et al. [33] were different, the effect on the protein was the same. Siggs and colleagues [34] also identified a large family with inherited autosomal nanophthalmos associated with a C-terminal frameshift variant in *MYRF* (c.3361delC, p.R1121Gfs36*) introducing a premature terminal codon in the penultimate exon. These familial cases of nanophthalmos are mostly non-syndromic, leading to the speculation that the ocular tissue is more sensitive to haploinsufficiency than the cardiac and urogenital tissues [6]. On the other hand, little is known so far about the function of the C-terminal part of MYRF located in the ER membrane.

In addition to the association between MYRF variants with congenital heart defects and nanophthalmos, Hamanaka et al. described *MYRF* as a new candidate gene for DSD [7], after a case-control study comparing gene-based burdens of rare damaging variants between both groups. The authors described four new *MYRF* variants in five individuals from four families. From those, three patients were 46,XY and two were 46,XX. All of them presented different phenotypes of DSD; however, only one had a diaphragmatic hernia, and neither heart defects nor nanophthalmos were associated in those patients. More recently, Globa et al. [8] reported two other cases of *MYRF* heterozygous variants as a cause of DSD. Both individuals were 46,XY; the first one registered as a female with ambiguous genitalia, later raised as a boy, and the second one was a girl with primary amenorrhea, a lack of secondary sexual characteristics and high-grade hypermetropia. According to the authors, the *MYRF* loss-of-function variant described in this patient was the first case combining gonadal dysgenesis and nanophthalmos phenotypes. Here, we present the case of a 46,XY patient with PGD, Scimitar syndrome, pulmonary vein malformation and severe hyperopia, who, to the best of our knowledge, is the first case involving eye, heart and genital defects due to a *MYRF* disruptive variant.

Although the function of this gene in sex development pathways is still unclear, the association of heterozygous de novo variants with gonadal dysgenesis in both 46,XY and 46,XX individuals points to an important function in early gonadal development [4,7]. Based on our bioinformatics analyses utilizing scRNA-seq, we bring robust evidence that *MYRF* is expressed mainly in cells of the coelomic epithelium during early development of the bipotential gonads. Similar results were reported by Hamanaka et al. in 2019, using a different scRNA data set, thus corroborating our results. The coelomic epithelium constitutes the first layer of cells in the urogenital ridge at the fourth week post fertilization (wpf), and during the fifth wpf they proliferate, forming a thickened multi-layered cluster of cells that differentiates into the primordial gonad or gonadal ridge. Some of the CE cells transform into NR5A1-positive gonadal precursors that later differentiate into Sertoli and granulosa cells, as well as into steroidogenic cells [35]. At the same time, the primordial germ cells migrate from the hindgut into the NR5A1-positive gonadal precursor cells [36,37]. CE cells have an important role in the early development of the bipotential gonads. Therefore, disrupting variants in the *MYRF* gene, which is highly expressed in this cell population, could have an impact in the normal development of the gonads.

Of the differentially expressed genes with a binding site for *MYRF*, *CITED2* (OMIM * 602937) caught our special attention. *CITED2* is involved in early gonadal development and sex determination. In mice, *Cited2* is expressed in the urogenital ridge and cooperates with *Wt1* to stimulate the transcription of *Nr5A1* [29,38]. In addition, a physical interaction of CITED2 and WT1 was shown by immunoprecipitation (IP), as well as GST pulldown, revealing an interaction with both WT1 isoforms ($^{+/-}$KTS) [38]. Buaas et al. had shown that CITED2 functions to ensure high expression levels from *Nr5a1 and Sry*, providing a proper activation of the male pathway during sex development, and providing evidence that *Sry* is a downstream target of the CITED2/WT1/NR5A1 regulatory pathway [29]. Moreover, reduced gene dosage of *Wt1* or *Nr5a1* in *Cited2* mutant gonads leads to partial sex reversal and can undergo complete XY sex reversal in the context of a hypomorphic *Sry* allele [29]. A transcriptional delay of male development in *Cited2*$^{-/-}$ mice was reported by Combes et al. [30], due to a reduction of *Nr5a1* levels at early gonadal development. Furthermore, XX *Cited2*$^{-/-}$ gonads showed defects in ovary differentiation with ectopic cell migration, transient upregulation of testis promoting factor *Fgf9* and delay of ovary promoting genes *Wnt4* and *Foxl2*, suggesting *Nr5a1* as an ovarian promoting gene. Human variants in *CITED2*, such as in *NR5A1*, are associated with premature ovarian failure (POF) [39,40]. Our finding that, in humans, *CITED2* is found upregulated in *MYRF* positive cells of the coelomic epithelium of the ovaries and contains a *MYRF* binding site makes *MYRF* a potential candidate as a new upstream regulator of early gonadal development. Therefore, haploinsufficiency of this gene may lead to different forms of gonadal dysgenesis in 46,XX and 46,XY individuals, and *CITED2* might be an important downstream target of *MYRF*.

Interestingly, *CITED2* is also required for heart morphogenesis, as well as establishment of the left–right axis in humans and mice [31,41,42]. $Cited2^{-/-}$ mice die during gestation with diverse cardiovascular malformations, such as atrial and ventricular septal defects (ASD/VSD), aberrant aortic arches, and common arterial trunk and left–right patterning defects [31,42], a phenotype very similar to that of patients with heterozygous de novo variants in *MYRF*. In humans, variants in *CITED2* were identified in patients with congenital heart defects (CHD) such as sinus venosus atrial septal defects, abnormal pulmonary venous return to the right atria, Tetralogy of Fallot, dextrocardia and other ventricular septal defects [41,43], also seen in patients with *MYRF* variants [44]. More importantly, several of these variants are localized in the promoter region of *CITED2* and have been proven to alter *CITED2* transcriptional activity, decreasing their expression [41,45]. Therefore, it is possible that haploinsufficiency of transcription factors of *CITED2*, such as *MYRF*, can influence its expression levels and lead to heart defects.

It is also important to highlight that according to an in silico prediction of the genome aggregation database (gnomAD v2.1.1) *MYRF* is a constraint gene and the value of pLI (probability of being loss-of-function intolerant) is 1, supported by a very low LOEUF (loss-of-function observed/expected upper bound fraction) value of 0.117, which means that this is a haploinsufficient gene, where loss of a single copy is not tolerated [46]. This is corroborated by the finding that, such as in our case, de novo variants are associated with most of the syndromic forms. In contrast, familiar cases of nanophthalmos are mostly associated with variants in the last exon, and other features of the CUGS are only seen in some individuals [6,33,34]. In the same way, no loss-of-function variants have been observed so far in *CITED2* in gnomAD, making *CITED2* a potential candidate of a downstream factor of *MYRF* whose reduced expression may induce the observed phenotypes in humans. Haploinsufficiency is frequently observed in cases of DSD produced by heterozygous variants or copy number variations in transcriptions factors such as *NR5A1*, *SOX9*, *NR0B1* or *WT1*, demonstrating that sex determination is highly sensitive to gene dosage [47–49]. Therefore, phenotypic variability of *MYRF* haploinsufficiency on gonadal development was expected since it acts in the same pathway. Nevertheless, further epigenetic and transcriptome studies in the respective gonadal and/or heart tissues will be necessary to elucidate the pleiotropic developmental effects of *MYRF* variants in the context of gene regulation and protein interaction.

5. Conclusions

Our data give evidence that heterozygous inactivating variants in *MYRF* may influence the upregulation of *CITED2* and thereby impact the *NR5A1* pathway of sex development very early in the gonadal ridge of both sexes, which might make *MYRF* haploinsufficiency a feasible cofactor disease due to missing upregulation of *CITED2*. Further investigations are needed to elucidate the interaction between *MYRF* and *CITED2*. In addition, a missing upregulation of *CITED2* by *MYRF* in heart development might also be the cause for abnormal pulmonary venous return to the right atria, atrial septal defect (ASD) or tetralogy of Fallot (ToF), as well as a left–right patterning defect that is observed in humans with heterozygous *CITED2* variants and $Cited2^{-/-}$ mice [31,41]. Heterozygous variants in *MYRF* are also associated with nanophthalmos. To our knowledge, we present the first case with a combination of three *MYRF* associated phenotypic features: heart defects (CHD, dextrocardia, anomalous pulmonary venous return), 46,XY PGD and severe hyperopia. A reason for this might be the very recent description of the CUGS, as well as the separate detection of C-terminal *MYRF* variants in familiar cases of nanophthalmos without further

CUGS symptoms and the different time points of diagnosis. While cardiac failures are detected at birth, nanophthalmos might be only detected during the first years of childhood, and gonadal dysgenesis is often only detected at puberty, all by different specialists, making a common diagnosis often difficult.

Supplementary Materials: The following supporting information can be downloaded at: https://www.mdpi.com/article/10.3390/jcm11164858/s1, Figure S1: Heatmap of the mean expression value in each cell cluster of the marker genes used to identify the cell populations found in testes samples; Figure S2: Heatmap of the mean expression value in each cell cluster of the marker genes used to identify the cell populations found in ovaries samples; Figure S3: Violin plot showing *MYRF* gene expression values in each cell population. Each dot represents the normalized expression value of *MYRF* in a cell. Cell clusters with less than ten cells were discarded. Table S1: List of samples reanalysed in this study derived from previous publications and deposited in the Gene Expression Omnibus database (GEO).

Author Contributions: Conceptualization, R.W.; formal analysis, V.C.-S., A.K., H.B. and F.O.; investigation, R.W. and M.A.-S.; writing—original draft preparation, R.W., V.C.-S. and H.F.-S.; writing—review and editing, R.W., O.H., L.W. and H.B.; visualization, V.C.-S. and H.F.-S.; supervision, R.W. and H.B.; funding acquisition, O.H. and H.B. All authors have read and agreed to the published version of the manuscript.

Funding: This work was funded by financial support from Bundesministerium für Bildung und Forschung BMBF (01DQ17004) and Deutsche Forschungsgemeinschaft (DFG, German Research Foundation) under Germany's Excellence Strategy (EXC 22167- 390884018) and Bundesministerium für Gesundheit (BMG). V.C.-S. and O.H. have received funding by the German Ministry of Health (grant No. 2519FSB503) for the project "Standardized and centred care for DSD over the lifespan (DSDCare)". H.F.-S. received a scholarship from Fundação de Amparo à Pesquisa do Estado de São Paulo (FAPESP #2020/13421-8) and by the Alexander von Humboldt Fellowship. M.A.-S. received a DAAD scholarship within the German Egyptian Research Long-term Scholarship (GERLS) Programme, 2019, No. 57460069. The funders had no role in study design, data collection and analysis, decision to publish, or preparation of the manuscript.

Institutional Review Board Statement: The study was conducted according to the guidelines of the Declaration of Helsinki and approved by the local Ethics Committee of the University of Lübeck (AZ08-081, AZ17-219).

Informed Consent Statement: Written informed consent including pseudonymised publication of scientific results was obtained from the parents/legal guardians of the patient.

Data Availability Statement: The data presented in this study were previously published and are openly available in NCBI's Gene Expression Omnibus [50], and are accessible through GEO Series accession number GSE143380 [20], GSE143356 [20], GSE124263 [17], GSE161617 [19] and GSE134144 [18].

Acknowledgments: V.C.-S., F.O., A.K. and H.B. acknowledge computational support from the OMICS compute cluster at the University of Lübeck.

Conflicts of Interest: The authors declare no conflict of interest.

References

1. Emery, B.; Agalliu, D.; Cahoy, J.D.; Watkins, T.A.; Dugas, J.C.; Mulinyawe, S.B.; Ibrahim, A.; Ligon, K.L.; Rowitch, D.H.; Barres, B.A. Myelin gene regulatory factor is a critical transcriptional regulator required for CNS myelination. *Cell* **2009**, *138*, 172–185. [CrossRef] [PubMed]
2. Koenning, M.; Jackson, S.; Hay, C.M.; Faux, C.; Kilpatrick, T.J.; Willingham, M.; Emery, B. Myelin gene regulatory factor is required for maintenance of myelin and mature oligodendrocyte identity in the adult CNS. *J. Neurosci. Off. J. Soc. Neurosci.* **2012**, *32*, 12528–12542. [CrossRef] [PubMed]
3. Bujalka, H.; Koenning, M.; Jackson, S.; Perreau, V.M.; Pope, B.; Hay, C.M.; Mitew, S.; Hill, A.F.; Lu, Q.R.; Wegner, M.; et al. MYRF is a membrane-associated transcription factor that autoproteolytically cleaves to directly activate myelin genes. *PLoS Biol.* **2013**, *11*, e1001625. [CrossRef] [PubMed]

4. Qi, H.; Yu, L.; Zhou, X.; Wynn, J.; Zhao, H.; Guo, Y.; Zhu, N.; Kitaygorodsky, A.; Hernan, R.; Aspelund, G.; et al. De novo variants in congenital diaphragmatic hernia identify MYRF as a new syndrome and reveal genetic overlaps with other developmental disorders. *PLoS Genet.* **2018**, *14*, e1007822. [CrossRef] [PubMed]
5. Jin, S.C.; Homsy, J.; Zaidi, S.; Lu, Q.; Morton, S.; DePalma, S.R.; Zeng, X.; Qi, H.; Chang, W.; Sierant, M.C.; et al. Contribution of rare inherited and de novo variants in 2871 congenital heart disease probands. *Nat. Genet.* **2017**, *49*, 1593–1601. [CrossRef] [PubMed]
6. Garnai, S.J.; Brinkmeier, M.L.; Emery, B.; Aleman, T.S.; Pyle, L.C.; Veleva-Rotse, B.; Sisk, R.A.; Rozsa, F.W.; Ozel, A.B.; Li, J.Z.; et al. Variants in myelin regulatory factor (MYRF) cause autosomal dominant and syndromic nanophthalmos in humans and retinal degeneration in mice. *PLoS Genet.* **2019**, *15*, e1008130. [CrossRef]
7. Hamanaka, K.; Takata, A.; Uchiyama, Y.; Miyatake, S.; Miyake, N.; Mitsuhashi, S.; Iwama, K.; Fujita, A.; Imagawa, E.; Alkanaq, A.N.; et al. MYRF haploinsufficiency causes 46,XY and 46,XX disorders of sex development: Bioinformatics consideration. *Hum. Mol. Genet.* **2019**, *28*, 2319–2329. [CrossRef]
8. Globa, E.; Zelinska, N.; Shcherbak, Y.; Bignon-Topalovic, J.; Bashamboo, A.; Msmall es, C.K. Disorders of Sex Development in a Large Ukrainian Cohort: Clinical Diversity and Genetic Findings. *Front. Endocrinol.* **2022**, *13*, 810782. [CrossRef]
9. Hughes, I.A.; Houk, C.; Ahmed, S.F.; Lee, P.A. Consensus statement on management of intersex disorders. *Arch. Dis. Child.* **2006**, *91*, 554–563. [CrossRef]
10. Capel, B. Vertebrate sex determination: Evolutionary plasticity of a fundamental switch. *Nat. Rev. Genet.* **2017**, *18*, 675–689. [CrossRef]
11. Elzaiat, M.; McElreavey, K.; Bashamboo, A. Genetics of 46,XY gonadal dysgenesis. *Best Pract. Res. Clin. Endocrinol. Metab.* **2022**, *36*, 101633. [CrossRef] [PubMed]
12. Stöhr, H.; Marquardt, A.; White, K.; Weber, B.H. cDNA cloning and genomic structure of a novel gene (C11orf9) localized to chromosome 11q12→q13.1 which encodes a highly conserved, potential membrane-associated protein. *Cytogenet Cell Genet* **2000**, *88*, 211–216. [CrossRef] [PubMed]
13. An, H.; Fan, C.; Sharif, M.; Kim, D.; Poitelon, Y.; Park, Y. Functional mechanism and pathogenic potential of MYRF ICA domain mutations implicated in birth defects. *Sci. Rep.* **2020**, *10*, 814. [CrossRef] [PubMed]
14. Li, H.; Durbin, R. Fast and accurate short read alignment with Burrows-Wheeler transform. *Bioinformatics* **2009**, *25*, 1754–1760. [CrossRef] [PubMed]
15. DePristo, M.A.; Banks, E.; Poplin, R.; Garimella, K.V.; Maguire, J.R.; Hartl, C.; Philippakis, A.A.; del Angel, G.; Rivas, M.A.; Hanna, M.; et al. A framework for variation discovery and genotyping using next-generation DNA sequencing data. *Nat. Genet.* **2011**, *43*, 491–498. [CrossRef]
16. Rausch, T.; Zichner, T.; Schlattl, A.; Stutz, A.M.; Benes, V.; Korbel, J.O. DELLY: Structural variant discovery by integrated paired-end and split-read analysis. *Bioinformatics* **2012**, *28*, i333–i339. [CrossRef] [PubMed]
17. Sohni, A.; Tan, K.; Song, H.W.; Burow, D.; de Rooij, D.G.; Laurent, L.; Hsieh, T.C.; Rabah, R.; Hammoud, S.S.; Vicini, E.; et al. The Neonatal and Adult Human Testis Defined at the Single-Cell Level. *Cell Rep.* **2019**, *26*, 1501–1517.e1504. [CrossRef]
18. Guo, J.; Nie, X.; Giebler, M.; Mlcochova, H.; Wang, Y.; Grow, E.J.; DonorConnect; Kim, R.; Tharmalingam, M.; Matilionyte, G.; et al. The Dynamic Transcriptional Cell Atlas of Testis Development during Human Puberty. *Cell Stem Cell* **2020**, *26*, 262–276.e264. [CrossRef]
19. Guo, J.; Sosa, E.; Chitiashvili, T.; Nie, X.; Rojas, E.J.; Oliver, E.; DonorConnect; Plath, K.; Hotaling, J.M.; Stukenborg, J.B.; et al. Single-cell analysis of the developing human testis reveals somatic niche cell specification and fetal germline stem cell establishment. *Cell Stem Cell* **2021**, *28*, 764–778.e764. [CrossRef]
20. Chitiashvili, T.; Dror, I.; Kim, R.; Hsu, F.M.; Chaudhari, R.; Pandolfi, E.; Chen, D.; Liebscher, S.; Schenke-Layland, K.; Plath, K.; et al. Female human primordial germ cells display X-chromosome dosage compensation despite the absence of X-inactivation. *Nat. Cell Biol.* **2020**, *22*, 1436–1446. [CrossRef]
21. Chen, S.; Zhou, Y.; Chen, Y.; Gu, J. fastp: An ultra-fast all-in-one FASTQ preprocessor. *Bioinformatics* **2018**, *34*, i884–i890. [CrossRef] [PubMed]
22. Melsted, P.; Booeshaghi, A.S.; Liu, L.; Gao, F.; Lu, L.; Min, K.H.J.; da Veiga Beltrame, E.; Hjorleifsson, K.E.; Gehring, J.; Pachter, L. Modular, efficient and constant-memory single-cell RNA-seq preprocessing. *Nat. Biotechnol.* **2021**, *39*, 813–818. [CrossRef] [PubMed]
23. Hao, Y.; Hao, S.; Andersen-Nissen, E.; Mauck, W.M., 3rd; Zheng, S.; Butler, A.; Lee, M.J.; Wilk, A.J.; Darby, C.; Zager, M.; et al. Integrated analysis of multimodal single-cell data. *Cell* **2021**, *184*, 3573–3587.e3529. [CrossRef] [PubMed]
24. Roselli, S.; Gribouval, O.; Boute, N.; Sich, M.; Benessy, F.; Attie, T.; Gubler, M.C.; Antignac, C. Podocin localizes in the kidney to the slit diaphragm area. *Am. J. Pathol.* **2002**, *160*, 131–139. [CrossRef]
25. Rudat, C.; Grieskamp, T.; Rohr, C.; Airik, R.; Wrede, C.; Hegermann, J.; Herrmann, B.G.; Schuster-Gossler, K.; Kispert, A. Upk3b is dispensable for development and integrity of urothelium and mesothelium. *PLoS ONE* **2014**, *9*, e112112. [CrossRef] [PubMed]
26. Richards, S.; Aziz, N.; Bale, S.; Bick, D.; Das, S.; Gastier-Foster, J.; Grody, W.W.; Hegde, M.; Lyon, E.; Spector, E.; et al. Standards and guidelines for the interpretation of sequence variants: A joint consensus recommendation of the American College of Medical Genetics and Genomics and the Association for Molecular Pathology. *Genet. Med. Off. J. Am. Coll. Med. Genet.* **2015**, *17*, 405–424. [CrossRef]

27. Pinz, H.; Pyle, L.C.; Li, D.; Izumi, K.; Skraban, C.; Tarpinian, J.; Braddock, S.R.; Telegrafi, A.; Monaghan, K.G.; Zackai, E.; et al. De novo variants in Myelin regulatory factor (MYRF) as candidates of a new syndrome of cardiac and urogenital anomalies. *Am. J. Med. Genet. Part A* **2018**, *176*, 969–972. [CrossRef]
28. Fishilevich, S.; Nudel, R.; Rappaport, N.; Hadar, R.; Plaschkes, I.; Iny Stein, T.; Rosen, N.; Kohn, A.; Twik, M.; Safran, M.; et al. GeneHancer: Genome-wide integration of enhancers and target genes in GeneCards. *Database* **2017**, *2017*, bax028. [CrossRef]
29. Buaas, F.W.; Val, P.; Swain, A. The transcription co-factor CITED2 functions during sex determination and early gonad development. *Hum. Mol. Genet.* **2009**, *18*, 2989–3001. [CrossRef]
30. Combes, A.N.; Spiller, C.M.; Harley, V.R.; Sinclair, A.H.; Dunwoodie, S.L.; Wilhelm, D.; Koopman, P. Gonadal defects in Cited2-mutant mice indicate a role for SF1 in both testis and ovary differentiation. *Int. J. Dev. Biol.* **2010**, *54*, 683–689. [CrossRef]
31. Weninger, W.J.; Lopes Floro, K.; Bennett, M.B.; Withington, S.L.; Preis, J.I.; Barbera, J.P.; Mohun, T.J.; Dunwoodie, S.L. Cited2 is required both for heart morphogenesis and establishment of the left-right axis in mouse development. *Development* **2005**, *132*, 1337–1348. [CrossRef] [PubMed]
32. Chitayat, D.; Shannon, P.; Uster, T.; Nezarati, M.M.; Schnur, R.E.; Bhoj, E.J. An Additional Individual with a De Novo Variant in Myelin Regulatory Factor (MYRF) with Cardiac and Urogenital Anomalies: Further Proof of Causality: Comments on the article by Pinz et al. *Am. J. Med. Genet. Part A* **2018**, *176*, 2041–2043. [CrossRef] [PubMed]
33. Xiao, X.; Sun, W.; Ouyang, J.; Li, S.; Jia, X.; Tan, Z.; Hejtmancik, J.F.; Zhang, Q. Novel truncation mutations in MYRF cause autosomal dominant high hyperopia mapped to 11p12-q13.3. *Hum. Genet.* **2019**, *138*, 1077–1090. [CrossRef] [PubMed]
34. Siggs, O.M.; Souzeau, E.; Breen, J.; Qassim, A.; Zhou, T.; Dubowsky, A.; Ruddle, J.B.; Craig, J.E. Autosomal dominant nanophthalmos and high hyperopia associated with a C-terminal frameshift variant in MYRF. *Mol. Vis.* **2019**, *25*, 527–534.
35. Stevant, I.; Kuhne, F.; Greenfield, A.; Chaboissier, M.C.; Dermitzakis, E.T.; Nef, S. Dissecting Cell Lineage Specification and Sex Fate Determination in Gonadal Somatic Cells Using Single-Cell Transcriptomics. *Cell Rep.* **2019**, *26*, 3272–3283.e3273. [CrossRef] [PubMed]
36. Piprek, R.P.; Kloc, M.; Kubiak, J.Z. Early Development of the Gonads: Origin and Differentiation of the Somatic Cells of the Genital Ridges. *Results Probl. Cell Differ.* **2016**, *58*, 1–22. [CrossRef] [PubMed]
37. Pelosi, E.; Koopman, P. Development of the Testis. In *Reference Module in Biomedical Sciences*; Elsevier: Amsterdam, The Netherlands, 2017; pp. 1–8.
38. Val, P.; Martinez-Barbera, J.P.; Swain, A. Adrenal development is initiated by Cited2 and Wt1 through modulation of Sf-1 dosage. *Development* **2007**, *134*, 2349–2358. [CrossRef]
39. Lourenco, D.; Brauner, R.; Lin, L.; De Perdigo, A.; Weryha, G.; Muresan, M.; Boudjenah, R.; Guerra-Junior, G.; Maciel-Guerra, A.T.; Achermann, J.C.; et al. Mutations in NR5A1 associated with ovarian insufficiency. *N. Engl. J. Med.* **2009**, *360*, 1200–1210. [CrossRef]
40. Fonseca, D.J.; Ojeda, D.; Lakhal, B.; Braham, R.; Eggers, S.; Turbitt, E.; White, S.; Grover, S.; Warne, G.; Zacharin, M.; et al. CITED2 mutations potentially cause idiopathic premature ovarian failure. *Transl. Res.* **2012**, *160*, 384–388. [CrossRef]
41. Sperling, S.; Grimm, C.H.; Dunkel, I.; Mebus, S.; Sperling, H.P.; Ebner, A.; Galli, R.; Lehrach, H.; Fusch, C.; Berger, F.; et al. Identification and functional analysis of CITED2 mutations in patients with congenital heart defects. *Hum. Mutat.* **2005**, *26*, 575–582. [CrossRef]
42. Bamforth, S.D.; Braganca, J.; Farthing, C.R.; Schneider, J.E.; Broadbent, C.; Michell, A.C.; Clarke, K.; Neubauer, S.; Norris, D.; Brown, N.A.; et al. Cited2 controls left-right patterning and heart development through a Nodal-Pitx2c pathway. *Nat. Genet.* **2004**, *36*, 1189–1196. [CrossRef] [PubMed]
43. Yang, X.F.; Wu, X.Y.; Li, M.; Li, Y.G.; Dai, J.T.; Bai, Y.H.; Tian, J. Mutation analysis of Cited2 in patients with congenital heart disease. *Zhonghua Er Ke Za Zhi* **2010**, *48*, 293–296. [PubMed]
44. Rossetti, L.Z.; Glinton, K.; Yuan, B.; Liu, P.; Pillai, N.; Mizerik, E.; Magoulas, P.; Rosenfeld, J.A.; Karaviti, L.; Sutton, V.R.; et al. Review of the phenotypic spectrum associated with haploinsufficiency of MYRF. *Am. J. Med. Genet. Part A* **2019**, *179*, 1376–1382. [CrossRef] [PubMed]
45. Zheng, S.Q.; Chen, H.X.; Liu, X.C.; Yang, Q.; He, G.W. Genetic analysis of the CITED2 gene promoter in isolated and sporadic congenital ventricular septal defects. *J. Cell Mol. Med.* **2021**, *25*, 2254–2261. [CrossRef] [PubMed]
46. Lek, M.; Karczewski, K.J.; Minikel, E.V.; Samocha, K.E.; Banks, E.; Fennell, T.; O'Donnell-Luria, A.H.; Ware, J.S.; Hill, A.J.; Cummings, B.B.; et al. Analysis of protein-coding genetic variation in 60,706 humans. *Nature* **2016**, *536*, 285–291. [CrossRef]
47. Werner, R.; Mönig, I.; August, J.; Freiberg, C.; Lünstedt, R.; Reiz, B.; Wünsch, L.; Holterhus, P.M.; Kulle, A.; Döhnert, U.; et al. Novel Insights in 46,XY Disorders of Sex Development due to NR5A1 Gene Mutation. *Sex. Dev. Genet. Mol. Biol. Evol. Endocrinol. Embryol. Pathol. Sex Determ. Differ.* **2015**, *9*, 260–280. [CrossRef]
48. Croft, B.; Ohnesorg, T.; Hewitt, J.; Bowles, J.; Quinn, A.; Tan, H.; Corbin, V.; Pelosi, E.; van den Bergen, J.; Sreenivasan, R.; et al. Human sex reversal is caused by duplication or deletion of core enhancers upstream of SOX9. *Nat. Commun.* **2018**, *9*, 5319. [CrossRef]
49. Eozenou, C.; Gonen, N.; Touzon, M.S.; Jorgensen, A.; Yatsenko, S.A.; Fusee, L.; Kamel, A.K.; Gellen, B.; Guercio, G.; Singh, P.; et al. Testis formation in XX individuals resulting from novel pathogenic variants in Wilms' tumor 1 (WT1) gene. *Proc. Natl. Acad. Sci. USA* **2020**, *117*, 13680–13688. [CrossRef]
50. Edgar, R.; Domrachev, M.; Lash, A.E. Gene Expression Omnibus: NCBI gene expression and hybridization array data repository. *Nucleic Acids Res.* **2002**, *30*, 207–210. [CrossRef]

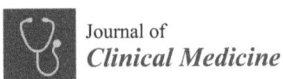

Article

Reassessment of Surgical Procedures for Complex Obstructive Genital Malformations: A Case Series on Different Surgical Approaches

Alice Hoeller [1,*], Sahra Steinmacher [1], Katharina Schlammerl [1], Markus Hoopmann [1], Christl Reisenauer [1], Valerie Hattermann [2], Sara Y. Brucker [1] and Katharina Rall [1,*]

[1] Department for Womens' Health, University of Tuebingen, 72074 Tübingen, Germany
[2] Department for Radiology, University of Tuebingen, 72074 Tübingen, Germany
* Correspondence: alice.hoeller@med.uni-tuebingen.de (A.H.); katharina.rall@med.uni-tuebingen.de (K.R.)

Abstract: The objective of this case series was to describe different uterus-preserving surgical approaches and outcomes in patients with complex obstructive Müllerian duct malformation caused by cervical and/or vaginal anomalies. A retrospective analysis was performed including patients undergoing uterovaginal anastomosis (n = 6) or presenting for follow-up (n = 2) at the Department for Gynecology at the University of Tuebingen between 2017 and 2022. Uterovaginal anastomosis was performed with a one-step combined vaginal and laparoscopic approach (method A), a two-step/primary open abdominal approach with primary vaginal reconstruction followed by abdominal uterovaginal anastomosis after vaginal epithelization (method B) or an attempted one-step approach followed by secondary open abdominal uterovaginal anastomosis due to reobstruction (method A/B). Patients presented at a mean age of 15 years. Two patients were treated by method A, four by method B and two by method A/B. Functional anastomosis was established in seven of eight patients, with normal vaginal length in all patients. Concerning uterovaginal anastomosis, the primary open abdominal approach with or without previous vaginal reconstruction seems to have a higher success rate with fewer procedures and should be implemented as standard surgical therapy for complex obstructive genital malformations including the cervix.

Keywords: obstructive Müllerian duct malformation; cervical aplasia; cervical atresia; hematometra; uterovaginal anastomosis

1. Introduction

Obstructive genital malformations including cervical agenesis/aplasia with or without transverse vaginal septum or (partial) vaginal aplasia belong to the group of complex Müllerian duct developmental disorders. In order to understand genital development disorders, it is essential to gain insight into the fundamentals of female embryological development. The genetic sex of each individual is determined by fertilization. In early embryological development (week 5–8), the mesonephric (Wolffian) and paramesonephric (Müllerian) ducts develop simultaneously. However, the presence of anti-Müllerian hormone (AMH), which is produced in the Sertoli Cells of the developing testis, disrupts the further development of the Müllerian duct in males. In absence of AMH, the Müllerian duct develops into the female phenotype, forming the uterus, cervix, fallopian tubes and the proximal part of the vagina. This process includes the elongation, fusion, canalization and partial resorption of the Müllerian duct. At approximately week 12 of gestation, the distal Müllerian duct fuses with the urogenital sinus, forming the vagina. Each of these steps is crucial for the unremarkable development of the female internal genitalia, and disruption at any point can cause different types of genital developmental disorders, including cervical agenesis or aplasia [1–3]. In general, Müllerian duct anomalies are described in 4–7% of the female population, although cases of cervical agenesis or aplasia (with or without a vagina) but with a functional uterus are rare [4–7].

Young women or girls often initially present with abdominal pain, primary amenorrhea and/or incapacity for sexual intercourse in cases of associated vaginal aplasia or thick transverse septum. In the long term, the incapacity for orthograde menstruation can result in hematometra/-kolpos with medical complications such as retrograde menstruation leading to endometriosis, organ adhesions, severe abdominal pain, infertility and infection. As a temporary solution, hormonal suppression of menstruation might be induced to prevent the reoccurrence of hematometra until a surgical strategy has been decided on or a functional uterovaginal anastomosis has been established. Such an approach can be reasonable for very young girls, as compliance with and understanding of therapy is essential. The limited surgical expertise and a lack of standardization with respect to the formation of a functional uterovaginal anastomosis or reformation of a functional cervix have historically led to hysterectomy as a radical surgical approach in young women or girls [8–10]. Nowadays, gynecological specialists seek not only to reduce morbidity but also to conserve the possibility of reproductive capacity. Therefore, there have been some reports describing surgical management [6,10,11]. In this article, we present different surgical approaches to uterus-conserving surgical therapy for different Mullerian anomalies performed at the Department for Women's Health of the University of Tuebingen, Germany, between 2017 and 2022.

2. Materials and Methods

This retrospective analysis included a total of 8 patients; 6 patients underwent surgery for uterovaginal anastomosis from 2017 to February 2022 at the Department for Women's Health of the University of Tuebingen, Germany. Two additional patients who presented at our outpatient clinic for genital malformations for follow-up examination within this period of time but had surgery performed in the years 2012 and 2015, respectively, were also included.

Mullerian duct anomalies were classified using the ESHRE/ESGE consensus classification system from 2013 (European Society of Human Reproduction (ESHRE) and Embryology-European Society for Gynaecological Endoscopy (ESGE) [5,12]. Patients included in this retrospective study presented with obstructive genital malformation due to cervical aplasia or atresia (C4), unilateral cervical aplasia (C3) and/or vaginal aplasia (V4) or transverse vaginal septum (V3).

Patient information concerning medical history, diagnosis, symptoms and treatment were obtained from medical records within the patient data system SAP GUI 7.70_DE as of January 2021. To depict the heterogenicity of the analyzed cases, a brief case report was summarized for each patient. Charts and tables were generated using Microsoft® Excel® 2019 and Microsoft® Word® 2019 (Redmond, WA, USA). Due to the descriptive character of the present study, no statistical tests were performed.

- Diagnostic and surgical strategy:

The diagnostic algorithm consisted of a thorough gynecologic examination, including the inspection of the vulva and, if possible, the vagina, vaginal and abdominal palpation; a vaginal, transabdominal or perineal 2D and 3D ultrasound; an MRI scan of the pelvis; and, when needed, laparoscopic validation of genital tract anomalies.

Patients with vaginal aplasia or thick obstructing proximal vaginal septum underwent treatment for neovagina/vaginal reconstruction following the modified McIndoe technique without a mesh graft, creating a vaginal canal by sharp and blunt dissection between the bladder and rectum [13–15]. Uterovaginal anastomosis was either laparoscopically established in a one-step procedure similar to the pull-through technique described elsewhere [16] (method A) or in a two-step/primary open abdominal procedure. In the latter cases, if necessary, a neovagina was first created as previously described or vaginal reconstruction/resection of vaginal septum was performed. After complete epithelialization of the neovagina, as a second step, a uterovaginal anastomosis was created using a combined vaginal and open abdominal approach similar to the push-trough method described elsewhere [16] (method B). Patients presenting with a normal vagina in width and length [17] were assigned to the two-step/open abdominal technique (method B) (Figure 1).

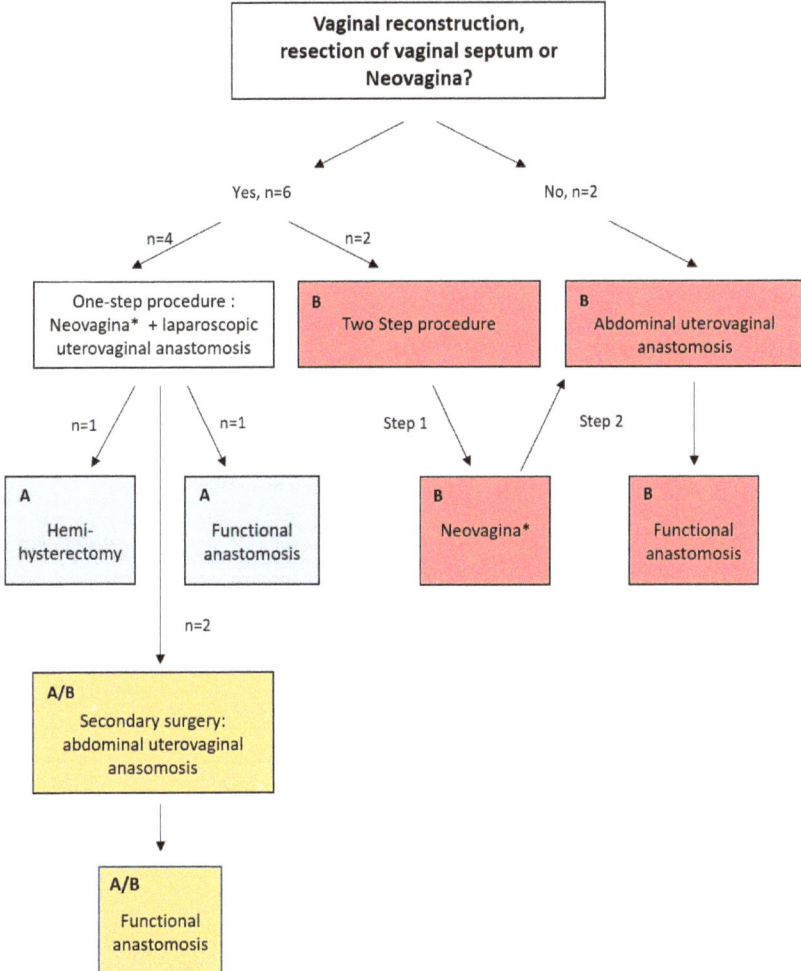

Figure 1. Surgical treatment algorithm. * Surgery for neovagina by modified McIndoe technique, vaginal reconstruction or resection of vaginal septum. (A) Method A: one-step creation of a neovagina* and simultaneous laparoscopic uterovaginal anastomosis procedure similar to the pull-through technique. (B) Method B: two-step/primary open abdominal technique: if necessary, creation of a neovagina* following a second-step open abdominal uterovaginal anastomosis similar to the push-through technique. (A/B): Method A/B: initial one-step technique analogous to method A and a secondary open abdominal uterovaginal anastomosis analogous to method B.

In the remaining cases, we initially attempted a single-step uterovaginal anastomosis, but after recurring stenosis/obstruction, uterovaginal anastomosis was established in an open abdominal approach (method A/B) similar to that adopted in method B. Patients presenting before 2017 were initially treated by method A, with the approach shifting toward method B after September 2019 as a result of surgical experience. The surgical treatment algorithm is shown in Figure 1. Ureters were preoperatively splinted prophylactically. Surgery was performed under a maximum of safety precautions, including vaginal, rectal and abdominal palpation and cystoscopy and intraoperative intravenous antibiotic application. Short-term outcomes were mostly evaluated in a secondary diagnostic hysteroscopy and/or gynecologic examination 4–6 weeks after surgery for uterovaginal anastomosis.

- Definition of outcome parameters:

Outcome measures were defined as follows:

1. Surgical outcome parameters:
   1.1 Primary surgical strategy
   1.2 Number of surgeries in total

   Diagnostic or, if required, unplanned surgery for the creation of a neovagina/vaginal reconstruction, uterovaginal anastomosis, planned follow-up examination with cervical dilation and hysteroscopy, recurrent cervical dilation, secondary uterovaginal anastomosis and other kinds of secondary surgery were performed.

2. Clinical outcome parameters concerning vagina and anastomosis
   2.1 Vaginal length and sexual intercourse;
   2.2 Orthograde menstruation;
   2.3 Sonographic exclusion of hematometra/-kolpos;
   2.4 Restenosis or reoccurring hematometra; and
   2.5 Complications.

3. Results and Presentation of Cases

3.1. Patient Characteristics

Patient characteristics are summarized in Table 1. Patients presented at a mean age of 15 years (range 11–20 years). Indications for clinical presentations at our department were either recurrent pelvic or abdominal pain due to hematometra or, in one case, pyometra, diagnostics for primary amenorrhea or the request for further treatment after diagnosis and/or treatment at another hospital.

There was one case of suspected OHVIRA (Obstructed hemivagina with ipsilateral renal anomaly) with bicorporal uterus (U3b) with unilateral cervical atresia (C3) and thick proximal transverse vaginal septum (case 1); three cases of hemiuterus (U4), either with (U4a; n = 2) or without (U4b; n = 1) rudimentary cavity; three cases of normal uterus (U0); and one case of dysmorphic T-shaped uterus (U1a). Complete cervical atresia (C4) was present in five cases, with cervix duplex (C3) in one case and two cases of patients with a normally configured cervix (C0) but vaginal aplasia (V4) or thick proximal transverse vaginal septum (V3). Vaginal aplasia (V4) was reported in two cases, with a transverse vaginal septum (V3) in two cases. In two cases, differentiation between thick vaginal septum and partial vaginal aplasia was not possible (V3/V4), and a normal vagina (V0) was observed in two cases (Table 1). Four of the eight patients presented with previously diagnosed associated malformations ranging from renal, skeletal, complex anogenital to cardiac defects. Five patients had been diagnosed with endometriosis genitalis externa.

Table 1. Patient characteristics.

Case Number	Age at Initial Presentation	ESHRE/ESGE	ASRM	Associated Malformations	Clinical Presentation	Endometriosis at Diagnosis
1	17	U3b C3 V3 / OHVIRA	Uterus didelphis R unilateral cervical agenesis Mid vaginal septum/OHVIRA	Unilateral renal aplasia right side	Hematometra	no

Table 1. Cont.

Case Number	Age at Initial Presentation	ESHRE/ESGE	ASRM	Associated Malformations	Clinical Presentation	Endometriosis at Diagnosis
2	13	U4a/C4/V4	R unicornuate uterus with L associated atrophic uterine remnant Cervical agenesis Distal vaginal agenesis	Multiple malformations: double kidney on both sides, skeletal malformations, anal atresia, tetralogy of fallot	Acute abdominal pain, pyometra	no
3	12	U4b C0 V3/4	L unicornuate uterus Normal cervix Distal vaginal septum	Renal agenesis right side	Abdominal pain	no
4	14	U4a C4 V3	R unicornuate with L associated atrophic uterine remnant Cervical agenesis Distal vaginal agenesis	Arterial septum defect and venticel septum defect, Arteria lusoria, konnatal hypothyroidism	Recurrent hematometra after surgery in other clinic	no
5	16	U0 C0 V4	Normal uterus Normal cervix Distal vaginal agenesis	-	Assumed vaginal septum, primary amenorrhea	yes
6	20	U0 C4, V0	Normal Uterus Cervical agenesis Normal vagina	-	Request for treatment, diagnosis at other clinic	yes
7	17	U1a C4 V3/4	T-shaped uterus Cervical agenesis Distal vaginal agenesis	-	Primary amenorrhea	yes
8	11	U0 C4 V0	Normal Uterus Cervical agenesis Normal vagina	-	Primary amenorrhea, pelvic pain	yes

ESHRE/ESGE: European Society of Human Reproduction (ESHRE) and Embryology-European Society for Gynaecological Endoscopy (ESGE); OHVIRA: Obstructed hemivagina with ipsilateral renal anomaly; ASRM: American Society for Reproductive Medicine.

3.2. Surgical Outcome Parameters

Surgery was performed at the Department for Women's Health of the University of Tuebingen, Germany. Each Surgery for uterovaginal anastomosis was performed by a team of at least two gynecologists with expertise in vaginal, laparoscopic and open abdominal surgery specialized in female genital malformations; one of the gynecologists was present at every operation. The continuity of the surgical team ensured that the outcome was not altered by expertise or surgical abilities.

The surgical strategy is visualized in Figure 1, and surgical outcome parameters are summarized in Table 2. In six of eight patients, surgical treatment for neovagina was achieved using the modified McIndoe technique, or vaginal reconstruction/resection of vaginal septum was performed. In four cases, a neovagina was created in a single-step technique in combination with uterovaginal anastomosis (Cases 1–4). Two patients were treated by method A, four by method B and two by method A/B (Figure 1). The total number of surgeries ranged from 3 to 11. Planned follow-up surgery by means of hysteroscopy and cervical dilation examination was performed in six of the eight cases. Secondary surgery was required in cases 1–4. Patients treated with method A had a mean number of 6.5 surgeries, patients treated by method B had a mean number of 3.75 surgeries and patients treated with method A/B had an average of 9 surgeries (Table 2).

Table 2. Surgical outcome parameters.

Case Number	ESHRE/ESGE	Treatment Algorithm	Diagnostic Surgery	Prior Surgery for Neovagina *	Date of Uterovaginal Anastomosis	Number of Surgeries for Uterovaginal Anastomosis	Planned Follow-Up Hysteroscopy And Cervical Dilation	Unplanned Hysteroscopy and Cervical Dilation	Secondary Surgery	Unplanned Hysteroscopy and Cervical Dilation	Total Number of Surgeries
1	U3b C3 V3/OHVIRA	A	0	no	28 April 2015	1	2	0	3	1	7
2	U4a/C4/V4	A	1	no	1 February 2012	1	0	0	1	3	6
3	U4b C0 V3/4	A/B	2 **	no	15 January 2015 15 September 2020	2	1	0	1	5	11
4	U4a C4 V3	A/B	0	no	July 2017 9 July 2019	2	1	1	2	1	7
5	U0 C0 V4	B	0	yes	2 March 2021	1	1	3	0	0	5
6	U0, C4, V0	B	1 **	no	2 February 2022	1	1	0	0	0	3
7	U1a C4 V3/4	B	2 ***	yes **	16 February 2022	1	1	0	0	0	4
8	U0 C4 V0	B	2	no	27 September 2017	1	0	0	0	0	3

OHVIRA: Obstructed hemivagina with ipsilateral renal; * Surgery for neovagina by modified McIndoe technique, vaginal reconstruction or resection of vaginal septum; ** surgery in other hospital, *** one diagnostic surgery in another hospital. (A) Method A: one-step creation of a neovagina * and a simultaneous laparoscopic uterovaginal anastomosis procedure similar to the pull-through technique. (B) Method B: two-step/open abdominal technique and, if necessary, creation a neovagina * following a second-step abdominal uterovaginal anastomosis similar to the push-through technique. (A/B): Method A/B: initial one-step technique analogous to method A, with secondary abdominal uterovaginal anastomosis. Planned follow-up surgery: cervical dilation and sometimes removal of a catheter or tube and hysteroscopy. Minor follow-up surgery: cervical dilation or hysteroscopy. Secondary surgery: procedures other than hysteroscopy and cervical dilation.

3.3. Clinical Outcome Parameters

Details are summarized in Table 3. All patients had a normal vaginal length > 6 cm [17], and three patients reported having had satisfying sexual intercourse.

Table 3. Clinical outcome parameters.

Case Number	Date of Uterovaginal Anastomosis	Latest Examination	Vaginal Lenght	Sexual Intercourse	Orthograde Menstruation	Absence of Hematometra	Re-Stenosis and/or Hematometra	Hysterectomy	Complications
1	28 April 2015	7 January 2019	n *	lost to follow up	normal menstruation normal left sided hemi uterus and cervix	yes, but pyometra right uterus	recurrent pyometra right hemiuterus	right sided hemi-hysterectomy, preserving the left-sided functional hemiuterus	-
2	26 January 2012	29 October 2018	n *	satisfying	yes, regular cycle	yes	yes, 3 × surgery for vaginal and/or cervical dilation, pyokolpos, sactosalpinx	-	-
3	15 January 2015 15 September 2020	11 April 2021	n *	satisfying	no, hormonal therapy	yes	recurrent vaginal discharge	-	-
4	July 2017 9 July 2019	14 March 2022	n *	not to date	yes	yes	-	-	-
5	2 March 2021	3 January 2022	n *	not to date	pending	yes	yes, 3 × dilation	-	-
6	2 February 2022	15 March 2022	n **	satisfying	pending	yes	pelvic pain and hematormetra after weaning from hormonal contraception	-	-
7	16 February 2022	22 March 2022	n **	not to date	pending	yes	-	-	-
8	27 September 2017	30 October 2017	n **	lost to follow up	lost to follow-up	yes	-	-	-

n = normal; * >6 cm counted as normal vaginal length [17]; ** no surgical intervention.

The absence of hematometra as an outcome parameter for functionality of uterovaginal anastomosis was achieved in all patients, although there was one case of recurrent pyometra, leading to hemi-hysterectomy and preserving the functional hemiuterus (case 1). Both patients treated by method A reported regular menstruation, with one patient menstruating out of the normally functioning hemiuterus (Case 1). One patient treated by method A/B reported regular menstruation, whereas the other patient did not menstruate under progesterone-only pill for contraception. The menstrual history of the four patients treated with method B is unknown/pending; one patient was lost to follow-up, and three patients had only received surgical treatment within the last three months of writing this article. Reasons for secondary surgery were reoccurrence of cervical or vaginal stenosis and/or reobstruction. Among all patients, there was the one case of hemi-hysterectomy, as mentioned above (case 1). No other complications occurred apart from the need for re-surgery due to stenosis and/or obstruction. To date, there has been no reported case of pregnancy.

3.4. Presentation of Cases

3.4.1. One-Step Approach, Method A

- Case 1

A 17-year-old girl presented in April 2015 with symptomatic advanced hematometra and partial hematokolpos. Clinical examination and ultrasound showed a bicorporal uterus with hematometra of the right side with suspected cervical hypoplasia and thick proximal vaginal septum with proximal hematokolpos on the right side. The left cervix and uterus seemed to be unaffected (ESHRE/ESGE classification: U3b C3 V3). Furthermore, the patient showed an aplasia of the right kidney; therefore, OHVIRA (obstructed hemivagina with ipsilateral renal anomaly) syndrome was suspected. Old blood was drained after dissection of the thick horizontal vaginal septum and reconstruction of the vagina with a method similar to the pull-through technique described by Bijsveldt et al., [16] thereby creating a uterovaginal anastomosis. Hysteroscopy of both hemiuteri was unsuspicious, although the right cervix could not be clearly detected. To prevent adhesions and closure, a Foley catheter was placed within the anastomosis. On the 8th day after surgery, the Foley catheter was replaced by a Fehling tube. One month later, the Fehling tube was removed, and cervical dilation was conducted. In August 2015, approximately 3 months after the primary surgery, the patient presented with recurrent hematometra on the right. Cervical dilation, hysteroscopy and diagnostic laparoscopy were performed, and again, a Foley catheter was placed into the cervix. The catheter was removed 5 days later, and the cervix was fixated by sutures. Due to recurrent hematometra on the right and physiological function of the left uterus, in October 2015, a right-sided supracervical hemihysterectomy was performed laparoscopically. With vaginal examination under general anesthesia prior to hysterectomy, we were not able to detect the previously reconstructed right cervix. The patient presented for follow up 1 month and 3 months after hysterectomy. She was asymptomatic and menstruated regularly, and the vaginal length was described as unsuspicious. Sonography showed minimal retention of fluid in the region of the previously formed right cervix. In July 2016, the patient was admitted due to abdominal pain and sonographically suspected with a hematocervix of 52 × 29 × 32 mm. Cervical mucus relief was obtained by laparoscopic incision. Again, the right-sided cervicovaginal anastomosis was not patent, cervical dilation was performed and a Fehling tube was inserted. Due to recurrent mucocervix, the cervix was surgically removed in December 2018. No further consultations at our department have taken place since then.

- Case 2

A 13-year-old girl presented with acute abdominal pain; therefore, emergency laparoscopy was performed. In addition to the medical history of multiple malformations such as bilateral double kidneys, skeletal malformations, anal atresia and tetralogy of fallot—for which surgery had been performed previously—laparoscopy showed vaginal and cervical atresia with a considerably enlarged right-sided hemiuterus and a rudimentary left uterine horn (ESHRE/ESGE classification: U4a/C4/V4), as depicted in Figure 2. After transfundal incision, pus was discharged. Then, a neovagina was created using the modified McIndoe procedure, and within the same surgery, a vaginally assisted laparoscopic uterovaginal anastomosis was established and a catheter was placed to contain the anastomosis. Five days later, the catheter was removed, and hysteroscopy and laparoscopy and reconstruction of the cervix were performed. A Fehling tube was inserted into the newly formed cervix, and the patient was instructed to use a vaginal stent at night. One month later, in March 2012, although the Fehling tube was still in the correct position within the uterovaginal anastomosis with no sign of hematometra, the vagina had obliterated completely and had to be reopened. Although a cervical formation had been performed in earlier surgeries, a cervix could not be identified. The Fehling tube was left within the anastomosis, and a vaginal device was placed into the vagina. Two months later, the patient presented for the removal of the vaginal device and Fehling tube. The neovagina was completely epithelialized and showed no sign of adhesions. However, the previously created cervix could now be identified as such. Aside from a small cervical polyp, hysteroscopy showed a normal cervical canal and hemiuterus. Follow-up examinations 1 and 3 months later showed no sign of hematometra, and menstruation occurred regularly. In November 2012, the patient was admitted due to pyometra for antibiotic and surgical treatment. The vagina had obliterated to a length of 2 cm, and the cervix was constricted. After dilation, pus discharged from the uterus. Vaginal reconstruction was performed, and a vaginal phantom was inserted. Follow-up examinations showed no sign of hematometra, and regular menstruation was achieved under oral hormonal contraceptive therapy. In September 2013, the patient was admitted again for therapy of pyometra. Laparoscopy and hysteroscopy showed advanced adhesions, which were cleaved. Follow-up 3 months later showed no sign of hemato- or pyometra, although menstruation was temporarily suppressed by hormonal therapy. The last presentation at our clinic was in 2018; menstruation occurred regularly, sexual intercourse was satisfying with a vaginal length of 7 cm and there was no sign of hemato- or pyometra.

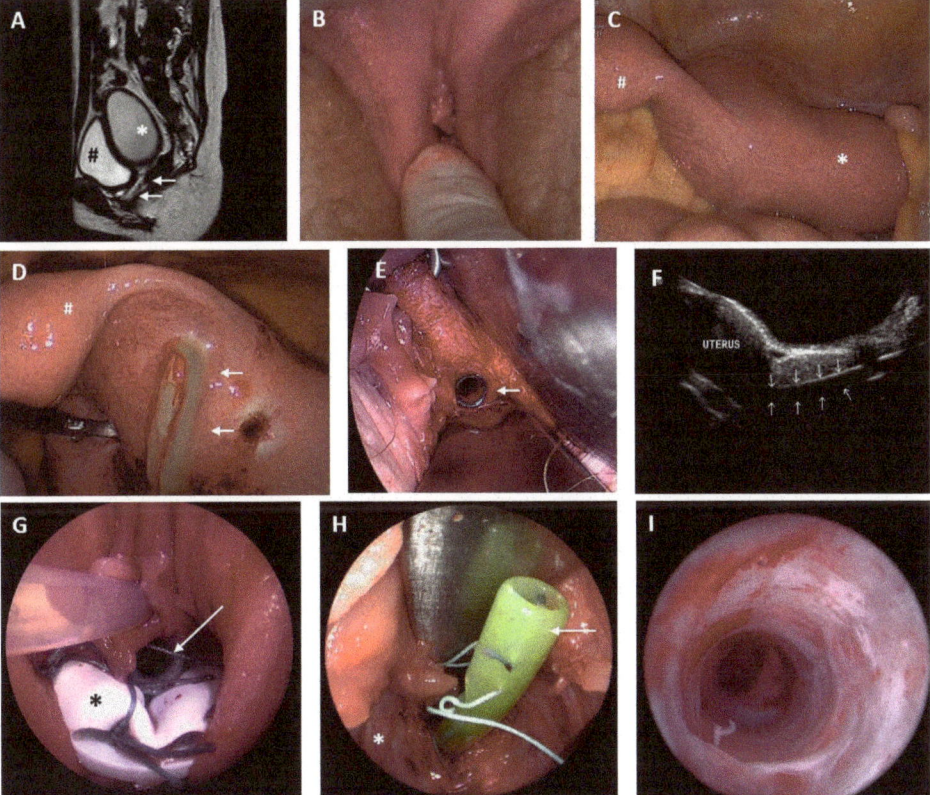

Figure 2. Case 2. (**A**) Magnetic resonance imaging from the pelvis; * hematometra (6.5 × 6.1 × 8.6 cm); arrows show vaginal atresia; # bladder. (**B**) Introitus vagina with vaginal atresia. (**C**) Laparoscopic view of an enlarged right-sided uterus unicornis (*) and a rudimentary left uteral horn (#). (**D**) Discharge of pus after transfundal incision (arrows); # left rudimentary uteral horn. (**E**) Arrow shows intracervical Fehling tube after vaginal and cervical reconstruction. (**F**) Transabdominal sonography; the uterus is displayed with normal endometrium on the left side; the right side of the picture, the intracervical Fehling tube is indicated by small arrows. (**G**) Vaginal device (*) with intracervical Fehling tube (arrow). (**H**) Fehling tube within the uterovaginal anastomosis (arrow), completely epithelialized neovagina (*). (**I**): Latest hysteroscopy after relief of pyometra and cleavage of adhesions.

3.4.2. One-Step Approach with Secondary Abdominal Uterovaginal Anastomosis Due to Reobstruction, Method A/B

- Case 3

A 12-year-old girl presented for further therapy after surgery was performed in another hospital due to severe abdominal pain with intraoperative diagnosis of partial vaginal aplasia or thick horizontal vaginal septum and hematometra with a left hemiuterus (ESHRE/ESGE classification: U4b C0 V3/4). Associated malformation: agenesis of right kidney. In January 2015, we performed surgery to create a neovagina using the modified McIndoe technique. The assumed cervix seemed to be dilated due to hematometra; further dilation and hysteroscopy were performed under laparoscopic view. To maintain uterovaginal anastomosis, a catheter was placed into the cervix. Five days later, the intrauterine catheter was removed, and the patient was instructed how to use a vaginal phantom. Six months later, vaginal shorting and cervical stenosis with recurrent hematometra was diagnosed, dilation was performed, and a catheter was inserted into the cervix again. After removal of the catheter hematometra reoccurred; therefore, hormonal therapy was started to suppress menstruation. In spite of hormonal suppression, in December 2015, hematometra had to be drained as a result of recurrent vaginal shortening and stenosis, and a stent was placed into the vagina. Hormonal suppression of menstruation was continued, and although vaginal shortening and stenosis reoccurred, the patient remained asymptomatic. In March 2020, the patient asked for vaginal reconstruction. Due to vaginal constrictions and adhesions with only mild hematometra and the absence of sexual activity, vaginal reconstruction was abandoned at that time. Hormonal therapy was stopped in order to develop hematometra, and surgery was scheduled in September 2020. Surgery was performed by a combined vaginal and open abdominal approach. The vagina was opened from the abdomen, and the recurrent vaginal stenosis was solved by a vaginal push-through anastomosis. Again, the patient was instructed how to use a vaginal phantom. Follow-up visits took place regularly; no further vaginal stenosis occurred, and cohabitation was possible without dyspareunia, with a vaginal length > 12 cm. No hematometra was documented, although the patient was under hormonal therapy; therefore, menstruation was suppressed temporarily. The latest visit at out department was in November 2021 due to excessive vaginal discharge probably caused by the long-lasting sutures, which was treated locally; otherwise, the patient did not have any complaints. Due to a progesterone-only pill for contraception, no menstruation was reported.

- Case 4

A 14-year-old girl presented with recurrent hematometra. The patient had been diagnosed with a bicorporal uterus with one cervix and a vaginal septum at another department of gynecology (ESHRE/ESGE classification: U4a C4 V3). Previous surgery at a different hospital: vaginal or hymenal incision and cervical dilation with discharge of hematometra and insertion of a catheter in the cervix. In a second-step vaginal reconstruction, laparoscopic removal of the left uterine horn had been performed, and a vaginal device and a Fehling tube were placed.

We initially performed surgery on the patient in March 2018. The vagina was nearly completely constricted; therefore, laparoscopic transfundal drainage of the hematometra was conducted. Then, a neovagina was reconstructed, and a vaginal device was put in place. Surgery for uterovaginal anastomosis was delayed until the vagina had healed completely; therefore, suppression of menstruation was initiated by hormonal therapy. With recurrent hematometra, in July 2019, vaginally assisted abdominal uterovaginal anastomosis was performed, and a catheter was placed into the anastomosis. One month later, vaginal dilation and dilation of the uterovaginal anastomosis was performed due to stenosis, and the patient was instructed to use a vaginal device again. In the following months, the patient presented regularly for follow-up, the vagina showed a circular stenosis with a length of 3–4 cm and menstruation was normal without signs of hematometra. In July 2021, 2 years after abdominal uterovaginal anastomosis, dilation of the uterovaginal anastomosis was necessary. The latest follow up was in March 2022; the patient showed no signs of hematometra, with a normal vaginal length and no signs of vaginal or uterovaginal stenosis.

3.4.3. Two-Step/Open Abdominal Approach, Method B

- Case 5

A 16-year-old asymptomatic girl presented with primary amenorrhea and suspected transverse vaginal septum or partial vaginal aplasia in October 2019. Physical examination showed an estimated vaginal length of 3 cm and no evidence of hematometra or -kolpos. Laparoscopy showed a normally configured uterus, intrabdominal adhesions and endometriosis genitalis externa (ESHRE/ESGE classification: U0 C0 V4). A neovagina was created using the modified McIndoe technique. Seventeen months after the successful creation of a neovagina, a cervicovaginal anastomosis was formed by vaginally assisted Pfannenstiel laparotomy similar to the push-through technique. A catheter was inserted into the newly created anastomosis. On the 6th postoperative day, the catheter was removed. The patient was instructed to insert a vaginal device. Within the next 8 months, five minor surgical interventions were performed for resolution of cervical stenosis. The last follow-up examination in January 2022—10 months after cervicovaginal anastomosis—showed a normal vaginal length and no signs of hematometra; however, menstruation was not reported since December 2021. Hormone analysis was unremarkable, and the endometrial thickness was 13 mm. At that time, surgical intervention was not indicated, and follow-up was recommended after 3–6 months or in case of any problems.

- Case 6

A 20-year-old woman presented with a surgically assured diagnosis of cervical aplasia/atresia and endometriosis (ESHRE/ESGE classification: U0 C4 V0). At presentation, the patient was under medication with a progesterone-only pill. The patient was asymptomatic, and physical examination showed no sign of hematometra, with a normal vaginal length (9–11 cm). In preparation for surgery, the patient was weaned from hormonal medication and subsequently developed abdominal pain and hematometra (Figure 3). Surgery for uterovaginal anastomosis was performed by Pfannenstiel laparotomy using the push-through technique and resection of the atretic cervical tissue in February 2022 (Figure 3). The previously described endometrioses was no longer detected. Follow-up surgery was scheduled after 6 weeks, comprising a hysteroscopy without any sign of cervical stenosis (Figure 3). Further follow-up is anticipated in the future.

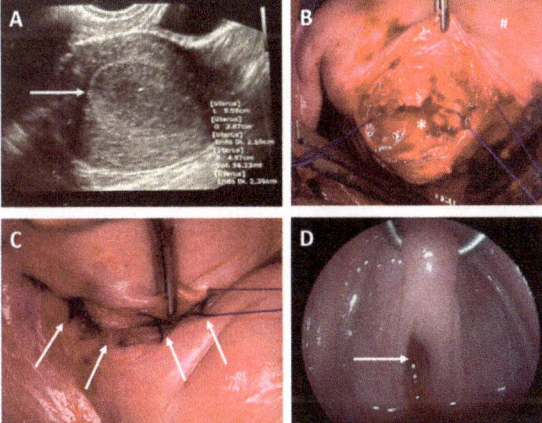

Figure 3. Case 6. (**A**) Transabdominal sonography; uterus with hematometra after weaning from hormonal therapy; arrows show significant hematometra. (**B**) Situs during abdominal laparotomy in preparation for uterovaginal anastomosis similar to the push-through technique; * transverse uterotomy after incision of the plica vesicouterina and caudal preparation of the bladder; # corpus uteri. (**C**) Circular, non-resorbable sutures; Prolene 2.0 establishing uterovaginal anastomosis (arrows). (**D**) Hysteroscopy shows open uterovaginal anastomosis (arrow) 6 weeks after initial surgery.

- Case 7

A 17-year-old patient presented with presumed genital malformation. Previously, the patient had undergone surgery for presumed vaginal septum, and a cervix could not be found. The patient had initially presented to her gynecologist at the age of 15 year with primary amenorrhea and moderate cyclic pain. The clinical examination depicted a vaginal length of 5–7 cm with a blind ending. An MRI scan suggested a T-formed uterus, cervical atresia, vaginal septum and enlarged ovaries with cysts on both sides (Figure 4). Diagnostic surgery was performed to identify the exact extent of genital malformation. Laparoscopically, endometriosis could be assured, the uterus presented with a T shape, the cervix uteri seemed to be absent and transverse vaginal septum or partial proximal vaginal aplasia was suspected (ESHRE/ESGE classification: U1a C4 V3/4). In February 2022, uterovaginal anastomosis via Pfannenstiel laparotomy using the push-through technique and resection of the atretic cervical tissue were performed, and a 14 Ch-silicon catheter was inserted into the cervix (Figure 4). Follow-up hysteroscopy and cervical dilation after 5 weeks showed a normal vaginal length with sufficient anastomosis and confirmed the presumed T-shaped uterus with no sign of infection. The next examination for follow-up is scheduled in July 2022.

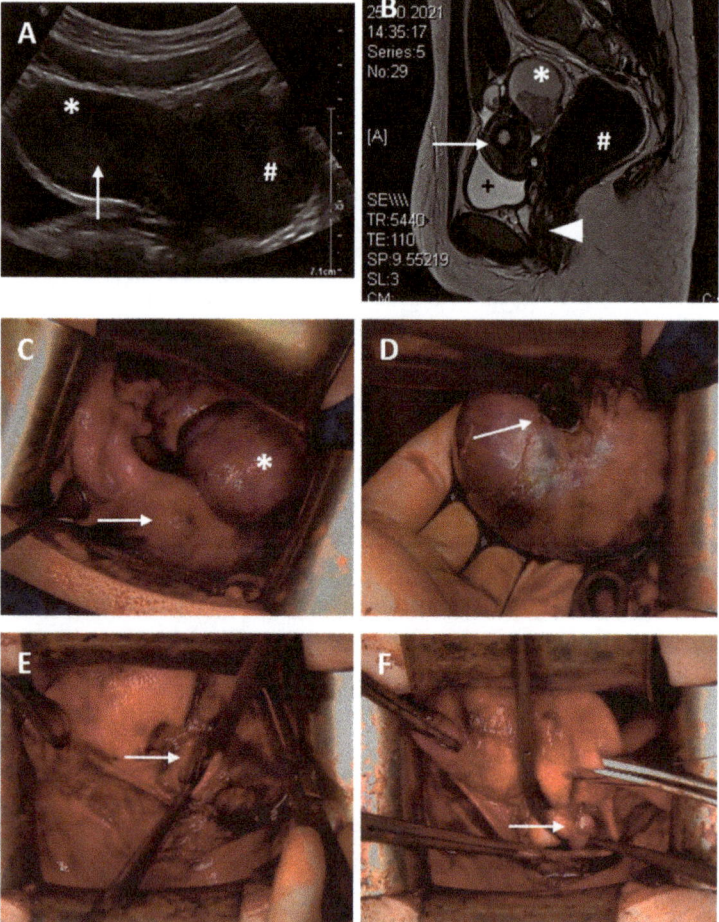

Figure 4. *Cont.*

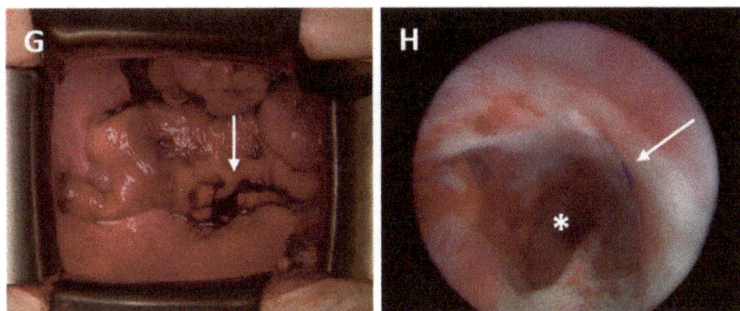

Figure 4. Case 6. (**A**) Transabdominal sonography; * uterus without hematometra; arrow depicts endometrium of 9 mm; # suspected rudimentary horn or myoma. (**B**) Abdominal magnetic resonance imaging: + full bladder, * suspected ovarian cyst 6 × 4 cm, # dilated rectum; arrow shows suspected T-shaped uterus without hematometra; arrowhead shows vagina; no connection from vagina to uterus. (**C**) Situs during abdominal laparotomy: arrow marks T-shaped uterus, * left side ovarian cyst of 10 cm diameter, suspicious for endometrioma (**D**) Incision of the suspected endometrioma and discharge of typical chocolate-like blood (arrow). (**E**): Insertion of an overhold clamp from the vagina (arrow) establishing a connection between the vagina and uterus. (**F**): Insertion of a 14 Ch-silicon catheter (arrow). (**G**) Uterovaginal anastomosis established by circular, non-resorbable Prolene 2.0 sutures (arrow). (**H**) Hysteroscopy after 5 weeks; sufficient uterovaginal anastomosis; * cavum uteri; arrow shows blue non-resorbable Prolene 2.0 suture.

- Case 8

An 11-year-old girl presented with severe abdominal pain and primary amenorrhea. Gynecological examination was performed under general anesthesia combined with diagnostic laparoscopy. The patient was found to have a vaginal length of 10 cm, but the cervix uteri was missing (ESHRE/ESGE classification: U0 C4 V0). Whereas the uterus appeared without hematometra or other abnormalities, a significant amount of blood was located in the abdomen, suggesting retrograde menstruation. Low-stage endometriosis was treated by coagulation. Due to the young age of the patient, hormonal therapy for suppression of menstruation was agreed upon. Regular follow-up was carried out in our outpatient clinic. At 14 years of age, the girl was admitted to hospital, and laparoscopy was performed because of severe abdominal pain and hematometra following reduced adherence to hormonal therapy. At 15 years of age, in September 2017, uterovaginal anastomosis was performed via Pfannenstiel laparotomy using the push-through technique, along with resection of the atretic cervical tissue, and a 14 Ch-silicon catheter was inserted into the newly formed anastomosis. The follow-up 4 weeks after surgery demonstrated an open cervix, and menstruation had not occurred, with no signs of hematometra or infection. The patient was then lost to follow-up.

4. Discussion

Due to the complex regulatory steps during Mullerian duct development, which include midline fusion, partial resorption and fusion with the urogenital sinus, development disorders can present in many different phenotypes. As identification of various types of obstructive Mullerian duct development is crucial for the success of surgical therapy, the combination of clinical examination, 2D and 3D ultrasound, MRI scanning of the pelvis and, in a second step, combined hysteroscopy and laparoscopy is the current diagnostic standard and should be performed before scheduling surgery for uterovaginal anastomosis [5,9].

In this case series, we describe eight cases of patients presenting with complex obstructive malformation including cervical aplasia or atresia with or without corresponding vaginal aplasia or thick proximal transverse vaginal septum. Unique medical histories with a diversity of symptoms or previously performed surgery make comparison of the cases difficult. Although discrimination between a thick proximal transverse vaginal septum and partial vaginal aplasia was not always possible [16], vaginal reconstruction and/or creation of a neovagina was necessary in both cases.

In four patients, a single-step vaginal reconstruction with simultaneous primary laparoscopy similar to the pull-through method for vaginal septum resection, if necessary, combined with cervical canalization or drilling, was performed to create a uterovaginal anastomosis [16,18]. Surgeries were performed between 2012 and 2017. In cases 3 and 4, recurrence of uterovaginal or vaginal stenosis led to secondary surgery similar to the abdominal push-trough method [16] for uterovaginal anastomosis in 2019 and 2020, respectively.

Cases 5–8 underwent primary surgery between 2017 and 2022. If creation of a neovagina, resection of vaginal septum or vaginal reconstruction was necessary, a two-step procedure was conducted. First, a neovagina was created, and only after completed epithelization of the vagina, uterovaginal anastomosis was constructed similar to the abdominal push-through technique. Formation of a neovagina or vaginal reconstruction was necessary in two cases; the other two cases had no pathology of the vagina [19,20] and an open abdominal uterovaginal anastomosis was created (step two of the two-step procedure) (Figure 1).

With increasing surgical experience and insufficient patency of uterovaginal anastomosis in a single-step laparoscopic approach (Cases 1, 3, 4), a drift to a two-step and open abdominal approach with assumed advantages might be proposed.

A long-term analysis by Deffarges et al. (2001) depicts similar results [21]. In our opinion, two main factors might play a role in the outcome.

First, patients with vaginal aplasia or thick transverse proximal vaginal septum and cervical aplasia require two surgical procedures consisting of the creation of a neovagina/vaginal reconstruction and the formation of a uterovaginal anastomosis. Both surgeries are complex procedures. The neovagina or reconstructed vagina has to heal, and occlusion is routinely prevented by the use of a vaginal and or cervical insert without a mesh graft [13,22,23]. When both steps of surgery are performed simultaneously, risk of occlusion or stenosis of the neovagina and uterovaginal anastomosis might be aggravated [9]. This might have accounted for cases 1, 3 and 4, in which a functional anastomosis failed to be established in a simultaneously vaginal reconstruction/creation of neovagina and laparoscopic uterovaginal anastomosis. Risk of vaginal reobstruction might be increased, as patients with obstructive genital malformations present at a young age, and compliance with the use of a vaginal phantoms or stents might not be optimal in comparison to older patients presenting for planned surgery for a neovagina, for example, in cases of MRKH [19,20,22].

Secondly, the main advantage of open abdominal uterovaginal anastomosis similar to the push-through technique, which was performed in the suggested two-step/open abdominal approach of cases 4–8, is the possibility of adequate creation and mobilization of the atretic cervix or uterus and its suture to the proximal vagina in a circular manner, forming a steady anastomosis using non-resorbable sutures. A similar approach was described by Grimbizis et al. (2004), whereas Kraim et al. (2020) used absorbable sutures, although the authors did not comment on the exact implementation of anastomosis [18,24]. Furthermore, if necessary, a cone can be resected if a fibrous cord or atretic cervix is present, as previously described [25,26]. This extent of uterine/cervical mobilization and visualization does not seem to be laparoscopically possible. Thus, in laparoscopic approaches a (re)canalization of an atretic cervix or fibrous cord was aspired, and attempts to avoid restenosis were made by using Foley catheters or Fehling tubes.

Regarding the year of primary surgery, within the analyzed collective at the Department for Women's Health of the University of Tuebingen, Germany, the primary surgical approach has changed from a single-step laparoscopic, to a one- or two-step open abdominal technique for uterovaginal anastomosis. This is in agreement with the current international recommendations [2,9,26].

Comparison of surgical strategies and the number of required surgeries is difficult, as literature is scarce and sole case reports are often presented [7,10,11,24,25,27,28]. Minami et al. (2019) described two cases of vaginal and cervical aplasia, which were successfully treated with the simultaneous creation of a neovagina using the modified McIndoe's technique (using an artificial skin graft) and either abdominal or laparoscopic creation of a uterovaginal anastomosis [11].

In patients with OHVIRA syndrome, a vaginal septum dissection is often sufficient, although hemi-hysterectomy has also been reported as a surgical solution, especially in cases of thick proximal vaginal septum, as in the case of our patient (case 1) [29,30].

Limitations of this analysis include the small sample size and the fact that the there had been no long-term follow-up for cases 6–8 to date due to the recent surgical therapy. Because many patients presented at young age, evaluation of sexual intercourse or pregnancies were inconclusive, and further follow-up is needed.

5. Conclusions

In conclusion, cases of obstructive genital malformations can be complex and heterogenous. Thus, individual approaches are necessary. The surgical two-step technique involving the creation of a neovagina or vaginal reconstruction in cases of thick transverse vaginal septum and the interval abdominally modified push-trough surgery for uterovaginal anastomosis seems to have advantages in terms of the overall outcome and should therefore be preferred. Adequate therapy has to be realized in specialized centers engaging multiprofessional teams.

Author Contributions: Conceptualization, A.H. and K.R.; Data curation, S.S., K.S. and C.R.; Formal analysis, A.H.; Funding acquisition, A.H.; Investigation, A.H.; Methodology, M.H., C.R. and S.Y.B.; Project administration, S.Y.B. and K.R.; Resources, S.Y.B. and K.R.; Supervision, K.R.; Visualization, M.H. and V.H.; Writing—original draft, A.H.; Writing—review & editing, K.S. and K.R. All authors have read and agreed to the published version of the manuscript.

Funding: This research was funded by the Open Access Publishing Fund of the University of Tuebingen.

Institutional Review Board Statement: The study was approved by the local ethics committee (Ethics Committee, Department of Medicine, Eberhard Karls University and University Hospital, Tuebingen, Germany; 779/2018BO2).

Informed Consent Statement: The patients consented to data and intraoperative pictures being generally used and published for research and teaching purposes. An additional written informed consent was not necessary due to the retrospective nature of this study.

Data Availability Statement: Patient information concerning medical history, diagnosis, symptoms and treatment were obtained from medical records within the patient data system SAP GUI 7.70_DE as of January 2021 from the Department for Women's Health of the University of Tuebingen, Germany.

Conflicts of Interest: The authors declare no conflict of interest. The funders (University of Tuebingen) had no role in the design of the study; in the collection, analyses, or interpretation of data; in the writing of the manuscript; or in the decision to publish the results.

Abbreviations

AMH: anti-Müllerian hormone; MRI: magnetic resonance imaging; OHVIRA: obstructed hemivagina with ipsilateral renal anomaly; ESGE: European Society for Gynaecological Endoscopy; ESHRE: European Society of Human Reproduction and Embryology; ASRM: American Society for Reproductive Medicine.

References

1. Reichman, D.E.; Laufer, M.R. Congenital uterine anomalies affecting reproduction. *Best Pract. Res. Clin. Obstet. Gynaecol.* **2010**, *24*, 193–208. [CrossRef] [PubMed]
2. Leitlinienprogramm der DGGG, OEGGG und SGGG 2018, Weibliche Genitale Fehlbildungen; AWMF Registernummer 015/052, Leitlinienklasse S2k, Stand 02/2020, Version 1.0. 2020. Available online: https://www.awmf.org/uploads/tx_szleitlinien/015-05 2l_S1_Weibliche_genitale_Fehlbildungen_2020-06.pdf (accessed on 19 June 2022).
3. Sadler, T.W. *Medizinische Embryologie*; Georg Thieme Verlag KG: Stuttgart, Germany, 2008; Volume 11, p. 529.
4. Santana Gonzalez, L.; Artibani, M.; Ahmed, A.A. Studying Mullerian duct anomalies—From cataloguing phenotypes to discovering causation. *Dis. Model Mech.* **2021**, *14*, dmm047977. [CrossRef] [PubMed]
5. Grimbizis, G.F.; Gordts, S.; Sardo, A.D.S.; Brucker, S.; De Angelis, C.; Gergolet, M.; Li, T.-C.; Tanos, V.; Brölmann, H.; Gianaroli, L.; et al. The ESHRE/ESGE consensus on the classification of female genital tract congenital anomalies. *Hum. Reprod.* **2013**, *28*, 2032–2044. [CrossRef]
6. Fujino, K.; Ikemoto, Y.; Kitade, M.; Takeda, S. Novel Method of Cervicoplasty Using Autologous Peritoneum for Cervicovaginal Atresia. *Surg. J.* **2020**, *6*, e28–e32. [CrossRef]
7. Roberts, C.P.; Rock, J.A. Surgical methods in the treatment of congenital anomalies of the uterine cervix. *Curr. Opin. Obstet. Gynecol.* **2011**, *23*, 251–257. [CrossRef]
8. Acien, P.; Acien, M.I. The history of female genital tract malformation classifications and proposal of an updated system. *Hum. Reprod. Update* **2011**, *17*, 693–705. [CrossRef]
9. Mikos, T.; Gordts, S.; Grimbizis, G.F. Current knowledge about the management of congenital cervical malformations: A literature review. *Fertil. Steril.* **2020**, *113*, 723–732. [CrossRef]
10. Rock, J.A.; Roberts, C.P.; Jones, H.W., Jr. Congenital anomalies of the uterine cervix: Lessons from 30 cases managed clinically by a common protocol. *Fertil. Steril.* **2010**, *94*, 1858–1863. [CrossRef] [PubMed]
11. Minami, C.; Tsunematsu, R.; Hiasa, K.; Egashira, K.; Kato, K. Successful Surgical Treatment for Congenital Vaginal Agenesis Accompanied by Functional Uterus: A Report of Two Cases. *Gynecol. Minim. Invasive Ther.* **2019**, *8*, 76–79.
12. Schöller, D.; Hölting, M.; Stefanescu, D.; Burow, H.; Schönfisch, B.; Rall, K.; Taran, F.-A.; Grimbizis, G.F.; Sardo, A.D.S.; Brucker, S.Y. Female genital tract congenital malformations and the applicability of the ESHRE/ESGE classification: A systematic retrospective analysis of 920 patients. *Arch. Gynecol. Obstet.* **2018**, *297*, 1473–1481. [CrossRef]
13. Marzieh, G.; Soodabeh, D.; Narges, I.-M.; Saghar, S.-S.; Sara, E. Vaginal reconstruction using no grafts with evidence of squamous epithelialization in neovaginal vault: A simple approach. *J. Obstet. Gynaecol. Res.* **2011**, *37*, 195–201. [CrossRef]
14. Banister, J.B.; McIndoe, A.H. Congenital Absence of the Vagina, treated by Means of an Indwelling Skin-Graft. *Proc. R. Soc. Med.* **1938**, *31*, 1055–1056. [CrossRef] [PubMed]
15. Wallwiener, D.J.W.; Kreienberg, R.; Friese, K.; Didrich, K.; Beckmann, M.W. *Atlas der Gynäkologischen Operationen*; Georg Thieme Verlag KG: Stuttgart, Germany, 2009; Volume 7.
16. van Bijsterveldt, C.; Willemsen, W. Treatment of patients with a congenital transversal vaginal septum or a partial aplasia of the vagina. The vaginal pull-through versus the push-through technique. *J. Pediatric Adolesc. Gynecol.* **2009**, *22*, 157–161. [CrossRef] [PubMed]
17. Lloyd, J.; Crouch, N.S.; Minto, C.L.; Liao, L.M.; Creighton, S.M. Female genital appearance: "normality" unfolds. *BJOG* **2005**, *112*, 643–646. [CrossRef] [PubMed]
18. Grimbizis, G.F.; Tsalikis, T.; Mikos, T.; Papadopoulos, N.; Tarlatzis, B.C.; Bontis, J.N. Successful end-to-end cervico-cervical anastomosis in a patient with congenital cervical fragmentation: Case report. *Hum. Reprod.* **2004**, *19*, 1204–1210. [CrossRef]
19. Rall, K.; Schenk, B.; Schäffeler, N.; Schöller, D.; Kölle, A.; Schönfisch, B.; Brucker, S.Y. Long Term Findings Concerning the Mental and Physical Condition, Quality of Life and Sexuality after Laparoscopically Assisted Creation of a Neovagina (Modified Vecchietti Technique) in Young MRKHS (Mayer-Rokitansky-Kuster-Hauser-Syndrome) Patients. *J. Clin. Med.* **2021**, *10*, 1269. [CrossRef]
20. Rall, K.; Schickner, M.C.; Barresi, G.; Schönfisch, B.; Wallwiener, M.; Wallwiener, C.W.; Wallwiener, D.; Brucker, S.Y. Laparoscopically assisted neovaginoplasty in vaginal agenesis: A long-term outcome study in 240 patients. *J. Pediatric Adolesc. Gynecol.* **2014**, *27*, 379–385. [CrossRef]
21. Deffarges, J.V.; Haddad, B.; Musset, R.; Paniel, B.J. Utero-vaginal anastomosis in women with uterine cervix atresia: Long-term follow-up and reproductive performance. A study of 18 cases. *Hum. Reprod.* **2001**, *16*, 1722–1725. [CrossRef]
22. Brucker, S.Y.; Gegusch, M.; Zubke, W.; Rall, K.; Gauwerky, J.F.; Wallwiener, D. Neovagina creation in vaginal agenesis: Development of a new laparoscopic Vecchietti-based procedure and optimized instruments in a prospective comparative interventional study in 101 patients. *Fertil. Steril.* **2008**, *90*, 1940–1952. [CrossRef]
23. Ellerkamp, V.; Rall, K.K.; Schaefer, J.; Stefanescu, D.; Schoeller, D.; Brucker, S.; Fuchs, J. Surgical Therapy After Failed Feminizing Genitoplasty in Young Adults With Disorders of Sex Development: Retrospective Analysis and Review of the Literature. *J. Sex. Med.* **2021**, *18*, 1797–1806. [CrossRef]
24. Kraiem, S.; Zoukar, O.; Hnayin, A.; Zouari, A.; Faleh, R.; Haddad, A. Complete cervical agenesis: Successful surgical treatment: One case report. *Pan Afr. Med J.* **2020**, *36*, 211. [CrossRef] [PubMed]
25. Jasonni, V.M.; La Marca, A.; Matonti, G. Utero-vaginal anastomosis in the treatment of cervical atresia. *Acta Obstet. Gynecol. Scand.* **2007**, *86*, 1517–1518. [CrossRef] [PubMed]

26. Zayed, M.; Fouad, R.; Elsetohy, K.A.; Hashem, A.T.; AbdAllah, A.A.; Fathi, A.I. Uterovaginal Anastomosis for Cases of Cryptomenorrhea Due to Cervical Atresia with Vaginal Aplasia: Benefits and Risks. *J. Pediatric Adolesc. Gynecol.* **2017**, *30*, 641–645. [CrossRef] [PubMed]
27. Gurbuz, A.; Karateke, A.; Haliloglu, B. Abdominal surgical approach to a case of complete cervical and partial vaginal agenesis. *Fertil. Steril.* **2005**, *84*, 217. [CrossRef] [PubMed]
28. Samantaray, S.R.; Mohapatra, I. Cervical Dysgenesis: A Rare Mullerian Duct Anomaly. *Cureus* **2021**, *13*, e18279. [CrossRef] [PubMed]
29. Romanski, P.A.; Bortoletto, P.; Pfeifer, S.M. Unilateral Obstructed Mullerian Anomalies: A Series of Unusual Variants of Known Anomalies. *J. Pediatric Adolesc. Gynecol.* **2021**, *34*, 749–757. [CrossRef]
30. Kudela, G.; Wiernik, A.; Drosdzol-Cop, A.; Machnikowska-Sokołowska, M.; Gawlik, A.; Hyla-Klekot, L.; Gruszczyńska, K.; Koszutski, T. Multiple variants of obstructed hemivagina and ipsilateral renal anomaly (OHVIRA) syndrome—One clinical center case series and the systematic review of 734 cases. *J. Pediatric Urol.* **2021**, *17*, 653.e1–653.e9. [CrossRef]

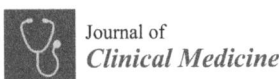

Article

Genome Sequencing and Transcriptome Profiling in Twins Discordant for Mayer-Rokitansky-Küster-Hauser Syndrome

Rebecca Buchert [1,†], Elisabeth Schenk [1,†], Thomas Hentrich [1], Nico Weber [2], Katharina Rall [3,4], Marc Sturm [1], Oliver Kohlbacher [2,5,6], André Koch [7], Olaf Riess [1,4], Sara Y. Brucker [3,4,†] and Julia M. Schulze-Hentrich [1,5,*,†]

1. Institute of Medical Genetics and Applied Genomics, University of Tübingen, 72076 Tübingen, Germany
2. Applied Bioinformatics, Department of Computer Science, University of Tübingen, 72076 Tübingen, Germany
3. Department of Women's Health, University of Tübingen, 72076 Tübingen, Germany
4. Rare Disease Center Tübingen, University of Tübingen, 72076 Tübingen, Germany
5. Institute for Bioinformatics and Medical Informatics, University of Tübingen, 72076 Tübingen, Germany
6. Institute for Translational Bioinformatics, University Hospital Tübingen, 72076 Tübingen, Germany
7. Research Institute for Women's Health, University of Tübingen, 72076 Tübingen, Germany
* Correspondence: julia.schulze-hentrich@med.uni-tuebingen.de; Tel.: +49-7071-29-72276
† These authors contributed equally to this work.

Abstract: To identify potential genetic causes for Mayer-Rokitansky-Küster-Hauser syndrome (MRKH), we analyzed blood and rudimentary uterine tissue of 5 MRKH discordant monozygotic twin pairs. Assuming that a variant solely identified in the affected twin or affected tissue could cause the phenotype, we identified a mosaic variant in *ACTR3B* with high allele frequency in the affected tissue, low allele frequency in the blood of the affected twin, and almost absent in blood of the unaffected twin. Focusing on MRKH candidate genes, we detected a pathogenic variant in *GREB1L* in one twin pair and their unaffected mother showing a reduced phenotypic penetrance. Furthermore, two variants of unknown clinical significance in *PAX8* and *WNT9B* were identified. In addition, we conducted transcriptome analysis of affected tissue and observed perturbations largely similar to those in sporadic cases. These shared transcriptional changes were enriched for terms associated with estrogen and its receptors pointing at a role of estrogen in MRKH pathology. Our genome sequencing approach of blood and uterine tissue of discordant twins is the most extensive study performed on twins discordant for MRKH so far. As no clear pathogenic differences were detected, research to evaluate other regulatory layers are required to better understand the complex etiology of MRKH.

Keywords: MRKH syndrome; monozygotic discordant twins; genome sequencing; transcriptome analysis; Müllerian ducts

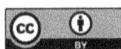

1. Introduction

Mayer-Rokitansky-Küster-Hauser (MRKH) syndrome is a rare congenital condition present in approximately one in 5000 live female births manifesting as aplasia or severe hypoplasia of structures related to the development of the Müllerian duct including the uterus and upper part of the vagina [1]. MKRH can either occur as an isolated form (type 1) or with additional extragenital phenotypes (type 2) such as renal or skeletal malformations [2]. Even though the occurrence of leiomyoma in women with MRKH is rare, multiple cases have been reported in the literature over the years, making it an important and easily overlooked differential diagnosis in MRKH patients presenting with abdominal pain [3,4]. Another difficulty women with MRKH face, is the inability to have sexual intercourse without previous neovagina surgery and to reproduce naturally. This can lead to severe psychological strain, further highlighting the importance of investigating this condition in more detail [5].

Females affected by MRKH syndrome usually have a normal 46.XX karyotype, normal ovarian function, and normal secondary sexual characteristics. In addition to various sporadic cases, several familial occurrences have been observed, suggesting a potential genetic origin of the syndrome [6]. Multiple genes have been subject to intensive investigation but could only partly be linked to a subset of MRKH cases in individual cohorts. Among them are genes essential for Müllerian and Wolffian duct development, which might play a key role in MRKH etiology [7]. Copy number variants (CNVs) in 1q21.1, 16p11.2, 17q12, and 22q11 with the corresponding genes *LHX1* and *HNF1B*, WNT signaling pathway genes such as *WNT4*, *WNT9B*, and the HOX family as well as some others have been pivotal candidates [8]. Recently, whole exome sequencing (WES) was used to identify *GREB1L* as a potential candidate for MRKH type 2 cases with kidney anomalies [9], but in general, the multifaceted and complex phenotype of the type 2 MRKH syndrome makes interpretation of genetic findings challenging. Until recently, previous work only focused on genome-wide CNV detection using array-CGH assays or WES and SNP arrays [10,11] limiting detection to exonic variants and therefore discarding potential mutations in regulatory factors. In 2019, Pan et al. [12] published results based on whole genome sequencing (WGS) for the detection of de novo variants in nine MRKH type 1 patients, which still remains, up to our knowledge, the only publication with a whole genome approach for MRKH patients complementing previously performed work.

As MRKH occurs mostly sporadically, this syndrome could also be explained by *de novo* dominant mutations in the germline of the offspring, or somatic mutations in the affected tissue. Those somatic variants, which might occur in early development, could also explain cases of monozygotic twins discordant for the MRKH syndrome [13–15]. Up until now, we are not aware of any publication analyzing and discussing tissue-specific variants in MRKH patients, which leads to certain unknowns concerning potential genetic mosaics in uterus rudiments as a potential source for MRKH type 1 and type 2 malformations.

To better understand the genetic contribution to MRKH etiology, we herein sequence and analyze the whole genome of blood and affected uterus rudiment of five twin pairs discordant for MRKH in an attempt to include regulatory features as well as potential tissue-specific gene alteration. In addition, we extend our tissue-specific endometrial transcriptome analysis from sporadic cases [16] to monozygotic discordant twins and evaluate perturbations in gene expression underlying MRKH.

2. Materials and Methods

2.1. Patients and Ethical Approval

From five MRKH-discordant pairs of MZ twins, blood samples, and clinical data were collected during routine clinical visits at the Department of Obstetrics and Gynecology, Tübingen University Hospital, Tübingen, Germany. The study was approved by the Institutional Review Board of the University of Tübingen (approval number: 205/2014BO1) and informed consent for genetic studies was obtained from each patient before recruitment.

Of the five patients with MRKH, one had type I and four had type II MRKH with associated renal malformations, one of whom had ureter abnormalities. Except for one pair, where both had renal agenesis, the corresponding co-twins were not affected by genital, renal, skeletal, or other malformations (Table 1). Tissue from uterine rudiments was collected from the affected twin during laparoscopic creation of a neovagina.

2.2. DNA Isolation and Sequencing

DNA from blood was isolated using the DNeasy purification kit and automated on the QIA-cube (Qiagen, Santa Clarita, CA, USA). DNA from rudimentary uterine tissue was isolated with the QiaAmp DNA Mini Kit (Qiagen). Genome sequencing was performed using the *TruSeq* PCR-free kit (Illumina, San Diego, CA, USA) on an Illumina platform (NovaSeq6000). Generated sequences were processed using the *megSAP* analysis pipeline (https://github.com/imgag/megSAP, accessed on 20 December 2021). *megSAP* performs quality control, read alignment, various alignment post-processing steps, variant detection, as well as comprehensive annotation of variants. Diagnostic analysis was performed using the *GSvar* clinical decision support system (https://github.com/imgag/ngs-bits, accessed on 20 December 2021). We used the GRCh38 reference genome assembly for the analysis.

Table 1. Phenotype of individuals in this study.

Twin Pair	Individual	Age at Surgery (Years)	Mrkh Type	Kidney Malformation	Skeletal Malformation	Heart Malformation	Vision
1	1-1	29	MRKH 2	Malrotation of kidney	Herniated disc	Fallot tetralogy	
2	2-1	19	MRKH 2	Kidney agenesis			Strabism
3	3-1	32	MRKH 2	Pelvic kidney			
3	3-2	-	-	Kidney agenesis	Hip dysplasia, scoliosis		
4	4-1	19	MRKH 1	-			
5	5-1	16	MRKH 2	Kidney agenesis			Strabism, poor vision

2.3. Genome Analysis and Variant Calling

The resulting data were then analyzed implementing different filter criteria and sample constellations.

Initially, the blood and tissue samples of the affected twins were compared to the respective healthy twin's blood samples using a multi-sample dominant filter (allele frequency < 0.10%, coding or near splice variants, keep pathogenic variants of HGMD or ClinVar, quality filter (quality: 250 | depth: 0 | mapq: 55 | strand bias: 20 | allele balance: 80)). We specifically searched for variants present in uterine tissue and blood of the affected twin, while absent in blood of the unaffected twin. Later, the multi-sample dominant filter was modified by including all coding or non-coding variants in MRKH target regions. This filter contained 612 regions and 752 different genes already described in the literature to be involved in uterine development and tissue genesis pathways.

The second analysis focused on comparing the affected twin's tissue and blood using once more the modified multi-sample dominant filter and target region filter.

Lastly, we analyzed for rare (<1% allele frequency) single nucleotide variants (SNVs), CNVs, or structural variants in the MRKH target region in the affected twin's tissue.

All remaining variants of the previous analyses were then manually evaluated, with respect to quality, conservation, the gene's biological functions, and previous association to MRKH.

2.4. Validation Using Sanger Sequencing

To validate the variant found in *ACTR3B*, primer pairs for Sanger sequencing were designed with Geneious Prime (Dotmatics, San Diego, CA, USA), a platform utilizing the widely used Primer3 algorithm. The resulting forward- (*ACTR3B*-F: TACTCTCAGGAG-GCTCCACC) and reverse-primer (*ACTR3B*-R: CCAGGGAGAGTGTGAAGCTG) were produced by metabion international AG (Steinkirchen, Germany). PCR was then performed using the Taq DNA Polymerase Kit (Qiagen, Santa Clarita, CA, USA) with a final volume of 40 µL containing 0.4 µL of Taq DNA Polymerase, 0.8 µL dNTPs, 4 µL QIAGEN PCR Buffer, 8 µL Q-Solution, 21.6 µL Ampuwa® (Fresenius, Bad Homburg, Germany), 2 µL genomic DNA (c = 36 ng/µL (blood samples); 110 ng/µL (tissue sample)) and 1.6 µL of each primer (10 µM). The resulting PCR amplicons were purified using the QIAquick® PCR Purification Kit (Qiagen, Santa Clarita, CA, USA) and later sequenced with the DCTS Quick Start Kit and CEQ™ 8000 Genetic Analysis System both by Beckman Coulter Inc. (Brea, CA, USA). All procedures were performed according to the manufacturer's manual.

2.5. RNA Isolation and Sequencing

Total RNA from the endometrium of rudimentary uterine tissue was isolated using the RNeasy Mini Kit (Qiagen) and used for paired-end RNA-seq. Quality was assessed with an Agilent 2100 Bioanalyzer (Santa Clara, CA, USA). Samples with high RNA integrity numbers (RIN > 7) were selected for library construction. Using the NEBNext Ultra II Directional RNA Library Prep Kit for Illumina and 100 ng of total RNA for each sequencing library, poly(A) selected paired-end sequencing libraries (101 bp read length) were generated according to the manufacturer's instructions. All libraries were sequenced on an Illumina NovaSeq 6000 platform at a depth of around 40 mio reads each. Library preparation and sequencing procedures were performed by the same individual, and a design aimed to minimize technical batch effects was chosen.

2.6. RNA Quality Control, Alignment, and Differential Expression Analysis

Read quality of RNA-seq data in fastq files was assessed using *FastQC* (v0.11.4) [17] to identify sequencing cycles with low average quality, adaptor contamination, or repetitive sequences from PCR amplification. Reads were aligned using *STAR* (v2.7.0a) [18] allowing gapped alignments to account for splicing against the *Ensembl* H. sapiens genome v95. Alignment quality was analyzed using *samtools* (v1.1) [19]. Normalized read counts for all genes were obtained using *DESeq2* (v1.26.0) [20]. Transcripts covered with less than 50 reads (median of all samples) were excluded from the analysis leaving 15,131 genes for determining differential expression. We set $|\log_2$ fold-change$| \geq 0.5$ and BH-adjusted *p*-value ≤ 0.05 to call differentially expressed genes. Gene-level abundances were derived from *DESeq2* as normalized read counts and used for calculating the $\log_2$-transformed expression changes underlying the expression heatmaps for which ratios were computed against mean expression in control samples. The *sizeFactor*-normalized counts provided by *DESeq2* also went into calculating nRPKMs (normalized reads per kilobase per million total reads) as a measure of relative gene expression [21]. Upstream regulators as well as predicted interactions among DEGs were derived from *Ingenuity Pathway Analysis* (IPA, v01–16, Qiagen). *Cytoscape* was used for visualizing networks [22]. Cell type-specific endometrial marker genes are based on single-cell data [23].

3. Results

3.1. Case Reports

For our study, we recruited five pairs of discordant monozygotic (MZ) twins of which one sister was affected with MRKH while the other sister did not show vaginal and uterus aplasia (Table 1). We obtained EDTA blood from both twins, their parents, as well as unaffected siblings willing to participate. We were also able to obtain tissue from the uterine rudiment of the affected twin (except twin 3). Additionally, kidney malformations were observed in four affected individuals (1-1, 2-1, 3-1, and 5-1), as well as the twin sister 3-2 who did not show features of MRKH. Additional phenotypic features such as skeletal, heart, or eye malformations were observed in three affected individuals (1-1, 2-1, and 5-1). In addition to twin sisters 3-2, none of the twins or siblings showed any of these additional phenotypes.

3.2. Multi-Sample Analysis of Twin Genomes for Discordant Variants

In the first analysis step, we performed multi-sample analyses of the blood and tissue of the affected twin against the blood of the unaffected twin as a control (Supplementary Tables S1 and S2). This filtering step gave us an average of 16 variants in the coding region, as well as seven variants in the non-coding regions. Since this filtering step enriched for technical artifacts, variant quality was assessed manually using IGV and resulted in only one mosaic variant of good quality in *ACTR3B* in twin 2 (Figure 1, Table 2). This variant (*ACTR3B* (ENST00000256001.13):c.1066G>A, p.Gly356Arg) had an approximate allele frequency of 39% in the affected tissue, 10% in the blood of the affected twin and only one read in the blood of the unaffected twin 2-2 (Figure 1). *ACTR3B* encodes a member of the actin-related proteins and plays a role in the organization of the actin cytoskeleton. It is highly expressed in the brain and many other tissues (https://www.proteinatlas.org/ENSG00000133627-ACTR3B/tissue, accessed on 15 February 2022). The glycine at position 365 is highly conserved and within the actin domain. Variants in *ACTR3B* have not been implied in MRKH or genitourinary malformation before and the functional consequences of this variant remain unclear.

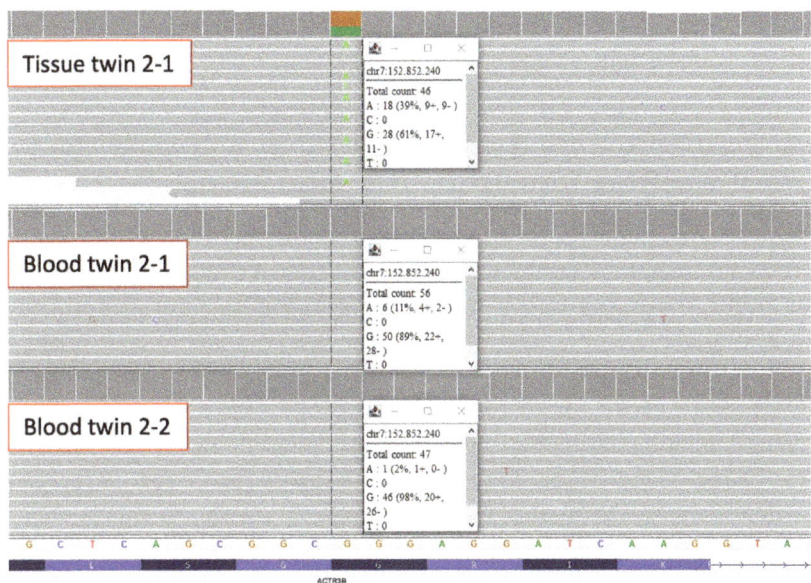

Figure 1. Mosaic missense variant in *ACTR3B* identified in blood and tissue of twin 2-1. IGV reads show that the variant c.1066G>A, p.Gly356Arg in *ACTR3B* has an allele frequency of about 39% in uterine tissue and an allele frequency of about 11% in blood of the affected twin 2-1, while blood of twin 2-2 only has 1 supporting read.

For the other twin pairs, a multi-sample analysis of tissue against the blood of the affected twin did not reveal any discordant variants.

Furthermore, we performed analyses for copy number variants and structural variants only present in the affected twin. Unfortunately, no variant with sufficient quality could be identified.

3.3. Analysis of Genome Data for Rare Conserved Variants in MRKH Candidate Genes

Under the assumption that the MRKH phenotype might not be fully penetrant, genome data were further analyzed for rare conserved single nucleotides as well as copy number or structural variants (Supplementary Table S3). This revealed one pathogenic variant in twin 3-1 (affected) and twin 3-2 (renal agenesis without features of MRKH), carrying a stop variant in *GREB1L* (ENST00000269218.10):c.4665T>A, p.Tyr1555* (Table 2). *GREB1L* is a target gene in the retinoic acid signaling pathway, which is highly expressed in the developing fetal human kidney and involved in the early metanephros and genital development [24]. Dominant variants in *GREB1L* have been previously described for renal hypodysplasia/aplasia 3 (OMIM #617805) including uterine abnormalities and MRKH. Interestingly, the twin sister not affected with MRKH had unilateral renal agenesis. Segregation analysis showed that this variant was inherited from a healthy mother. Reduced penetrance is well known for *GREB1L* variants [24,25]; thus, we classified this variant as pathogenic.

Table 2. Identified variants in SNV analysis.

Analysis Type	Sample	MRKHS Classification	Zygosity	Transcript (ENST-Number)	Variant Reads	Total Reads	Gene	cDNA Change	Protein Change	phyloP	gnomAD-Allele Frequency	Inheritance
Single sample analysis	Tissue MRKH-twin 1	MRKH-I	het	ENST00000263334.9	14	37	PAX8	c.1315G>A	p.Ala439Thr	42.050	0	AD
Single sample analysis	Tissue MRKH-twin 2	MRKH-I	het	ENST00000290015.7	20	31	Wnt9B	c.205C>T	p.Arg69Trp	27.030	0.0002180	AD
Single sample analysis	Tissue MRKH-twin 3	MRKH-II	het	ENST00000269218.10	33	51	GREB1L	c.4665T>A	p.Tyr1555Ter	-0.7730	0	AD
Multi sample analysis	Tissue MRKH-twin 2	MRKH-I	het	ENST00000256001.13	18	46	ACTR3B	c.1066G>A	p.Gly356Arg	75.720	0	AD
Multi sample analysis	Blood MRKH-twin 2	MRKH-I	het	ENST00000256001.13	6	56	ACTR3B	c.1066G>A	p.Gly356Arg	75.720	0	AD
	Blood healthy-twin 2	MRKH-I	wt		1	47	-	-	-	-	-	-

This table illustrates the SNVs found in the various analyses. The abbreveations are as follows: AD—autosomal dominant; het—heterozygous; n/a—not annotated; wt—wild type.

Furthermore, we identified a heterozygous *PAX8* variant (ENST00000263334.9: c.1315G>A, p.Ala439Thr) in twin 1-1 (affected), twin 1-2 (unaffected), as well as the unaffected mother (Table 2). *PAX8* has been postulated in MRKH before [7]. The variant affects a well-conserved amino acid within the paired-box protein 2C terminal domain of PAX8 and is not listed in gnomAD. According to ACMG criteria, we classified this variant as a variant of unknown significance.

In twin 2-1 (affected) and twin 2-2 (unaffected), a missense variant in *WNT9B* (ENST00000290015.7:c.205C>T, p.Arg69Trp) was detected which is also present in the unaffected sister and was inherited from the father (Table 2). Variants in *WNT9B* have been implicated in MRKH before [26,27]. This variant affects a conserved amino acid within the WNT domain and is listed in gnomAD [28] with a frequency of 0.0002. Among the individuals carrying this variant in gnomAD, there is no shift between female and male carriers. Nevertheless, we cannot exclude an effect of this variant on the MRKH phenotype potentially in combination with other variants. Thus, we classified this variant as variant of unknown significance.

3.4. MRKH Twins and Sporadic Cases Showed Largely Similar Endometrial Transcriptome Changes

To test whether the observed variants in *ACTR3B*, *GREB1L*, *PAX8*, and *WNT9B* altered their gene expression levels, we performed RNA-sequencing of uterine rudiments obtained from three affected twins (1-1, 2-1, and 4-1). Compared to previously published controls and sporadic MRKH patients [16], no significant change in gene expression was observed for these genes (Figure 2), indicating that the variants did not alter the underlying expression.

As discordant MRKH twins might be based on a distinct etiology when compared to sporadic cases, we next asked whether the overall endometrial transcriptome differs between discordant twins and sporadic cases. Therefore, we compared the three twin transcriptomes to previously published transcriptomes of 35 sporadic patients (19 type 1 and 16 type 2) as well as 25 controls [16]. Principal component analysis separated MRKH samples from controls and the three twin samples clustered together with those of sporadic cases, indicating a high similarity of transcriptomic signatures (Supplementary Figure S1). Based on single-cell data from endometrial tissue [23], cell type-specific expression of marker genes from ciliated and unciliated epithelial cells was highly similar between twins and sporadic cases (Supplementary Figure S2).

To compare these commonalities in more detail, differential expression changes were determined between MRKH twins and control samples. When compared to controls, a total of 449 differentially expressed genes (DEGs) with 235 being up- and 214 being down-regulated were identified (Figure 3A). Of those, 174 were also significantly changed in MRKH sporadic cases (Figure 3B), which in total included 2121 DEGs as previously reported [16]. Interestingly, 26 of the 174 DEGs showed opposing expression changes between twins and sporadic cases with the MZT twins appearing to be more similar to the expression pattern in controls than sporadic cases (Figure 3C, Supplementary Figure S3). These 26 DEGs were enriched for the Gene Ontology term *hydrolase activity* including genes such as *ATAD3B*, *CHTF18*, *HAGHL*, *HDAC10*, *PLA2G6*, and *RTEL1-TNFRSF6B*. However, the majority of the shared 174 DEGs showed largely similar expression changes in twins as well as sporadic samples when compared to controls (Figure 3C).

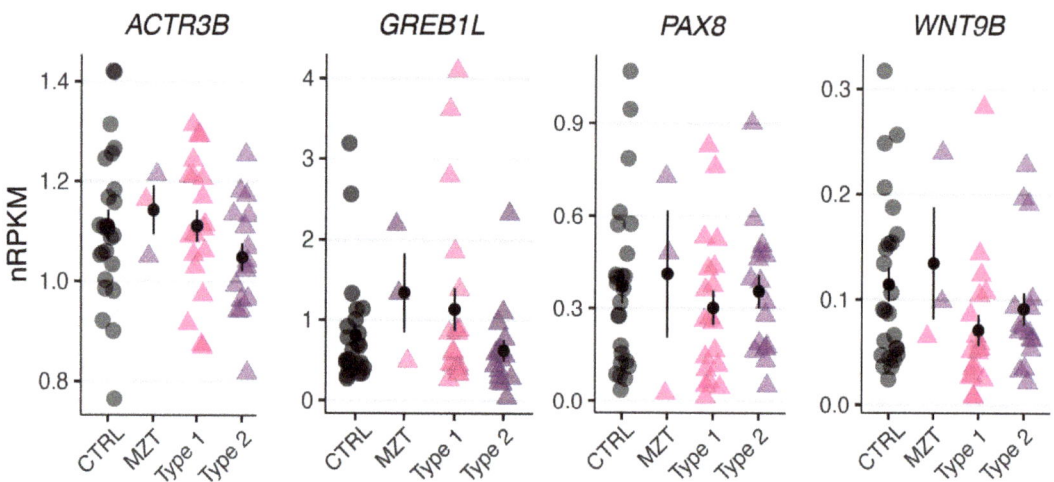

Figure 2. No significant change in genes expression observed for *ACTR3B*, *GREB1L*, *PAX8*, and *WNT9B*. Expression levels for the selected DEGs plotted as individual data points with mean ± SEM.

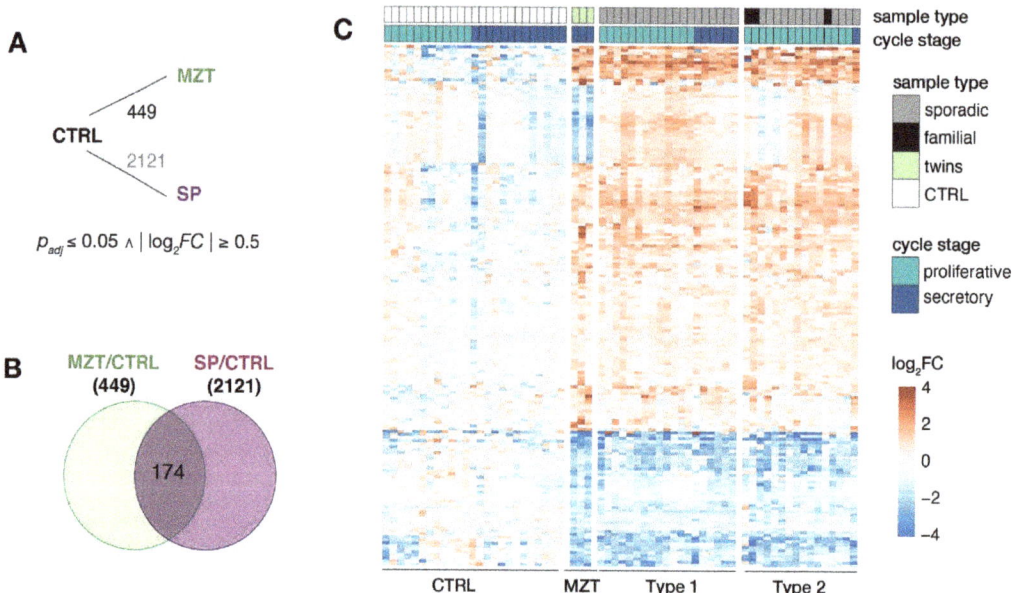

Figure 3. Endometrial transcriptomes of MRKH twins and sporadic cases show largely similar changes. (**A**) Schematic diagram of comparisons between MRKH monozygotic twins (MZT), MRKH sporadic cases (SP) and unaffected women (controls) indicating number of differentially expressed genes (DEGs). DEGs between sporadic cases and controls based on previous work [13]. Fold change and significance cut-offs below. (**B**) Venn diagram showing number of common DEGs MRKH twins and sporadic cases each compared to controls. (**C**) Expression profiles (log_2 expression change relative to *Ctrl* group) of 174 DEGs (common DEGs indicated in Figure 3B) across all samples. Rows hierarchically clustered by Euclidian distance and *ward.D2* method. Cycle information (proliferative or secretory) and patient type (monozygotic twin, sporadic, or control) on top.

To better understand the underlying biology of the endometrial perturbances in MRKH twins, enrichment analysis was then applied to identify molecules upstream of the observed DEGs. The most significant molecule observed was *fulvestrant* (Figure 4A), a selective estrogen receptor degrader (SERD), used as a medication to treat hormone receptor (HR)-positive metastatic breast cancer in postmenopausal women with disease progression as well as HR-positive, HER2-negative advanced breast cancer in combination with *palbociclib* in women with disease progression after endocrine therapy [29,30]. In line, the estrogen receptor itself was found as a significant upstream regulator (Figure 4A). Visualizing a network of DEGs around *fulvestrant* connects several key genes such as *WNT4* previously linked to MRKH (Figure 4B). Individually plotting gene expression changes of these candidates, further points to the similarity of endometrial gene expression changes between MRKH twins and sporadic cases (Figure 4C).

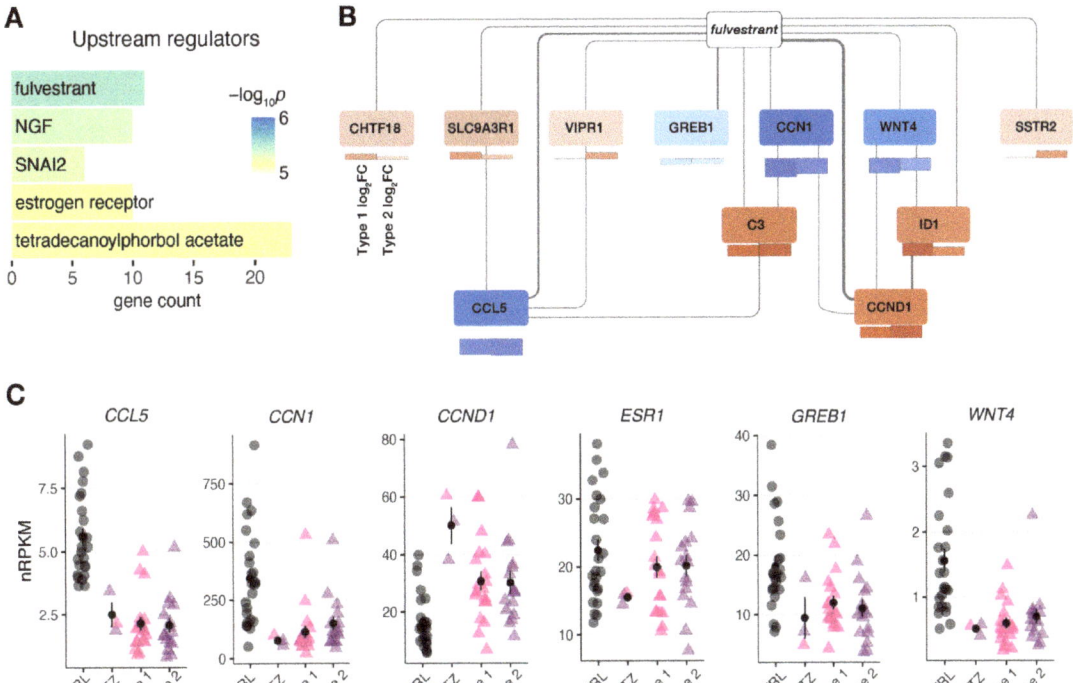

Figure 4. Gene expression changes in MRKH monozygotic twins point at regulators linked to estrogen receptor. (**A**) Predicted upstream regulators for common 174 DEGs (from Figure 3B) based on *Ingenuity Pathway Analysis*. Top five significant regulators shown. (**B**) Network of DEGs associated with upstream regulator *fulvestrant*. Interactions based on Ingenuity Pathway Analysis with line width indicating number of curated interactions. Genes color-coded by mean expression change observed in MZT/CTRL on top and SP/CTRL separately for type 1 and type 2 below. (**C**) Expression levels for the selected DEGs plotted as individual data points with mean ± SEM.

Taken together, our transcriptome analysis indicates that MRKH twins do not substantially differ from other MRKH cases and that, in general, observations made in twins can be transferred to sporadic cases as well.

4. Discussion

4.1. Etiology of MRKH Syndrome

The etiology of MRKH syndrome is complex, multifactorial and, to date, not well understood. Even though a number of candidate genes have been proposed, many lack functional evidence. Additionally, many familial cases show an autosomal dominant inheritance with incomplete penetrance and variable expressivity [6,31], which complicates genetic diagnosis using segregation analysis. Especially, missense variants in candidate genes are very hard to interpret in this context but also nonsense variants pose difficulties in this regard. While some studies showed that pathogenic loss of function variants in candidate genes such as *PAX8*, *BMP4*, and *BMP7* are predominantly inherited by the father [7], there is no sex difference seen for loss of function variants in gnomAD for these genes. This points towards reduced penetrance and further mechanisms involved in MRKH. Studying discordant twins poses an opportunity to investigate variants differing between the twins as well as looking for potential epigenetic marks and transcriptomic changes between these twins.

4.2. Genomic Differences of Monozygotic Twins

Even though monozygotic twins developed from the same zygote, they do not have the exact same genome. During development, a number of variants occur and may differ in variant allele frequency (VAF) between both twins depending on the timepoint and cell population of twinning. Some of these variants may be nearly constitutional with a VAF of >0.45, while others are mosaic with lower VAFs. A recent study of 381 monozygotic twins and two triplets estimated the average number of early developmental variants differing in twins to be around 5.2 [32]. The number of discordant variants observed for each twin pair had a huge variation ranging from more than 100 to no variant observed. In our study, we could only identify one mosaic variant in a total of five twin pairs and no nearly constitutional variant differing in the twins. One explanation could be that our cohort size is much smaller and may be biased towards a lower number of discordant variants. Another explanation could be that while we had average coverage of about 43×, the study by Jonsson and colleagues had coverage of 152× for many of their genomes leading to higher accuracy of variant and mosaic calling.

In a previous study, the same monozygotic twin pairs were analyzed using SNP arrays and potential CNVs of unknown clinical relevance were identified in affected twin 5-1 but not in her healthy sister [33]. These CNVs could not be replicated in this study. One reason for this could be the different methods applied. Recently, a study found that arrays sometimes produce artifacts, and genome data are more reliable for CNV calling (https://www.biorxiv.org/content/10.1101/2022.06.10.495642v1.full). Another reason for this discrepancy could be mosaic frequencies caused by analyzing DNA that was isolated from different parts of the affected tissue.

4.3. Mosaic Variant in ACTR3B

The only discordant variant we could identify in our twin cohort was a mosaic variant c.1066G>A, p.Gly356Arg in *ACTR3B*. *ACTR3B* encodes for an actin-related protein (ARP) involved in the organization of the cytoskeleton which has not been implied in MRKH or any other disorder so far. GTEx expression data for several tissues show a predominant expression of *ACTR3B* in the brain and a rather low expression in the uterus (https://www.proteinatlas.org/ENSG00000133627-ACTR3B/tissue, accessed on 15 February 2022). In contrast, protein levels of ACTR3B are relatively high in female tissue. During murine development, it is mainly expressed in embryonal ectoderm and not mesoderm or endoderm (derived from GXD [34]), which are more crucial to the development of the genital tract. *ACTR3B* is highly intolerant to loss of function variants with a pLI-score of 1 and the affected amino acid Gly356 is highly conserved within the actin domain. Still, without further functional evidence and the identification of further individuals with variants in *ACTR3B* and genitourinary anomalies, the connection between this mosaic variant and the observed phenotype remains elusive.

4.4. Pathogenic GREB1L Variant

Our analysis for rare conserved variants in candidate genes for MRKH identified a heterozygous loss of function variant c.4665T>A, p.Tyr1555* in *GREB1L*. *GREB1L* has been previously associated with a variety of genitourinary disorders (OMIM #617805) including MRKH [9,35–37]. Many affected families present with a pedigree with autosomal dominant inheritance and reduced penetrance and variable expressivity. This is also seen in the family presented here. The mother shows no symptoms of genitourinary malformations while one daughter has MRKH and a pelvic kidney (MRKH type 2) and her twin sister has unilateral kidney agenesis, hip dysplasia, and scoliosis with no evidence of MRKH. In previous reports on pathogenic *GREB1L* variants, the authors noted a bias in transmission towards maternal inheritance which might be caused by imprinting of the paternal allele [24,36]. The mothers transmitting the variant were usually unaffected or only showed a mild phenotype. This could also explain why the mother of twin pair 3 is unaffected but both her daughters show symptoms of *GREB1L* haploinsufficiency.

4.5. Variants of Unknown Significance

4.5.1. WNT9B

WNT9B encodes a secretory glycoprotein and paracrine factor that is part of the canonical Wnt signaling pathway, one of the main pathways responsible for the organization of the mammalian urogenital system by regulating embryonic development, adult tissue homeostasis, and differentiation [38]. In mice, it is mostly expressed in the developing kidney and epithelium of the Wolffian duct in both sexes, therefore playing an essential role in renal development [38].

Even though the gene is not highly expressed in the Müllerian duct, which later forms the uterus, oviduct, and upper part of the vagina, posterior Müllerian duct elongation is only made possible by Wnt9b mediated interactions with the epithelium of the Wolffian duct [38,39]. A study with *Wnt9b−/−* knock-out mice corroborates the above-mentioned mechanism, as males did not develop a vas deferens and epididymis and females lacked a uterus, oviduct, and upper vagina, whereas the gonads appeared normal, as is the case in MRKH [38].

Multiple studies found that some patients with Müllerian duct anomalies or MRKH did indeed have variants in *WNT9B* [26,27]. Furthermore, SNPs in this gene were linked to a higher MRKH risk [40]. However, a different study, comparing *WNT9B* variants of patients with Müllerian abnormalities to healthy controls, ruled out *WNT9B* variants as the only causative factor for Müllerian anomalies, as most of them could be found in a small number of healthy controls as well [41]. This phenomenon could also be observed in twin pair 2, which implies that WNT9B is not the only causative factor of MRKH, but might still be involved in its, yet to be understood, pathogenesis.

4.5.2. PAX8

The *PAX8* gene encodes a homeodomain signaling molecule, strongly expressed in the Müllerian duct, Wolffian duct, and kidney during embryonic development [42]. Together with *PAX2*, a gene closely related and partly redundant in function to *PAX8*, they initiate the mesenchymal–epithelial transition which later leads to the formation of the Wolffian duct [43]. The same mechanism is believed to be involved in the Müllerian duct formation [39]. Animal models corroborate this theory as *Pax2−/−* mice do not have kidneys nor a reproductive tract [43], only initially developing the anterior part of the Wolffian and Müllerian duct [44]. In *Pax2−/−Pax8−/−* embryos there is no Wolffian nor Müllerian duct formation at all.

The studies on *Pax8−/−* knock-out mice are quite controversial. Whereas Mittag et al. observed only remnants of myometrial tissue instead of a uterus and the absence of a vaginal opening in *Pax8−/−* mice [45], Mansouri et al. reported no urogenital malformations with the same knockout model [42]. Even if it is not yet clear whether a variant in *PAX8* alone is enough to disrupt urogenital development, the gene is certainly involved in this delicate process.

Furthermore, multiple *PAX8* variants and deletions have already been described in MRKH patients [7,46], indicating a connection between this gene and the MRKH pathogenesis.

4.6. Transcriptome Analysis of MRKH Twins

In addition to our genome analysis, we also used the chance to better understand gene expression perturbations in monozygotic twins and profiled the endometrial transcriptome of the affected twins. In contrast to a small subgroup of genes with opposing expression changes between twins and sporadic cases, the observed perturbations largely agreed with changes previously described in sporadic cases [16]. The main chemical associated with the shared DEGs was *fulvestrant*, a selective estrogen receptor degrader (SERD), used as a medication to treat hormone receptor (HR)-positive metastatic breast cancer in postmenopausal women with disease progression as well as HR-positive, HER2-negative advanced breast cancer in combination with *palbociclib* in women with disease progression after endocrine therapy [29,30]. In addition, the estrogen receptor itself was found as a significant upstream regulator and the gene encoding for estrogen receptor 1, *ESR1*, was perturbed in affected twins and sporadic cases in line with our previous findings [47–49].

Agreeing with previous literature, estrogens are necessary for the embryonic development of the female reproductive tract. The pivotal role of *ESR1* in female reproductive tract development has been previously shown by disrupting the corresponding gene in mice, subsequently leading to hypoplastic uterine and vaginal tissue [50]. Intriguingly, prenatal exposures of fetuses to synthetic estrogen such as diethylstilbestrol (DES) can also alter HOX gene expression in the developing Müllerian system, thereby disrupting the development of the female reproductive tract [51]. In the 1970s, DES was prescribed to pregnant women to prevent miscarriages until it was realized that daughters exposed to DES *in utero* showed a higher incidence of Müllerian anomalies [52] and a higher prevalence of MRKH [53].

Taken together, our transcriptome analysis confirms previous transcriptome perturbations in MRKH and points to high similarity of endometrial gene expression changes between twins and sporadic cases.

5. Conclusions

In this study, we examined the genetic differences of discordant twins as well as blood and affected tissue for MRKH using genome sequencing. To our knowledge, no previous study conducted genome sequencing for discordant MRKH twins or on the affected tissue. Even though our intention was to shed light on the genetic causes of MRKH by thoroughly checking for small copy number variants or structural variants missed by previous array analysis as well as identifying potential pathogenic variants in intronic, intergenic regions and non-coding transcripts, we were not able to identify any such causes neither in tissue nor as discordant variants nor as variants in candidate regions. One explanation for this could be the problem of interpreting such variants. Still, with our approach of sequencing discordant twins and more than one tissue, we were not able to identify a discordant variant in non-coding regions, indicating that it is more complex than just the interpretation of the variants in question. Another possibility would be that even after decades of deciphering the genome, some genomic regions are still not correctly mapped due to their highly repetitive nature. With our short-read genomes, we would not have been able to identify changes in these regions but would rather need long-read genome sequencing. Furthermore, our findings support the claim that MRKH is likely not inherited in a dominant fashion, which has also been observed in a study evaluating the frequency of congenital anomalies in biological children of MRKH patients [54]. The aforementioned study found that none of the 17 examined female children of MRKH mothers inherited the syndrome [54]. To summarize, MRKH patients do not appear to directly pass on the congenital condition to their children and as a general genetic cause has, to our knowledge, not yet been identified, the risk of MRKH occurring in biological daughters of affected women is small. The only clearly pathogenic variant we were able to identify was a loss of function variant in *GREB1L*. This shows that most likely previous studies of exome sequencing of blood did not miss out on a significant portion of pathogenic genetic variants. One explanation could be that the etiology of MRKH is far more complex, and incomplete penetrance, as seen for example in TAR syndrome [55], and variable expressivity hamper the identification of causative variants. The phenotypic discordance in the twins could also be explained by possible tissue mosaicisms not detected in this study. Another reason is that genetics might play a minor role in the development of MRKH and epigenetic changes as well as environmental and microbiological factors should be taken more into account when looking into the etiology of MRKH.

Supplementary Materials: The following supporting information can be downloaded at: https://www.mdpi.com/article/10.3390/jcm11195598/s1, Figure S1: Both MRKH twin and sporadic samples separated from control tissue in unaffected individuals; Figure S2: Gene expression of cell type-specific markers is similar between MRKH twins, sporadic cases, and unaffected controls; Figure S3: Subgroup of genes showing opposing expression changes between MRKH twins and sporadic cases.

Author Contributions: R.B. and E.S. performed the genome analysis and variant interpretation. R.B. and E.S. validated variants using Sanger sequencing. T.H. and J.M.S.-H. performed the bioinformatic analysis of RNA-sequencing data. K.R. and S.Y.B. obtained patient samples and were responsible for the clinical input. A.K. processed these samples. J.M.S.-H., S.Y.B., O.K. and O.R. conceived and designed the project. N.W. and M.S. set-up the analysis pipeline. R.B, E.S. and J.M.S.-H. wrote the manuscript with input from all authors. All authors have read and agreed to the published version of the manuscript.

Funding: This study was supported by a project grant of the Deutsche Forschungsgemeinschaft (DFG 351381475; BR 5143/5-1, AOBJ: 639534; KO 2313/7-1, AOBJ: 639535; RI 682/15-1, AOBJ: 639536) and through funding of the NGS Competence Center Tübingen (NCCT-DFG, project 407494995). JMS-H was supported by the *solveRD* consortium (European Union's Horizon 2020 research and innovation program under Grant Agreement No. 779257).

Institutional Review Board Statement: The study was approved by the Institutional Review Board of the University of Tübingen (approval number: 205/2014BO1).

Informed Consent Statement: Informed consent for genetic studies was obtained from each patient before recruitment.

Data Availability Statement: Genome and RNA-sequencing data that support the findings of this study have been deposited in the European Genome-phenome Archive (EGA) (primary accession number: EGAS00001006370, EGAS00001006371).

Acknowledgments: We thank all patients who participated in the study. We thank the team of the NGS Competence Center Tübingen, foremost Nicolas Casadei and Sven Poths, for their support.

Conflicts of Interest: The authors declare no competing interests.

References

1. Herlin, M.K.; Petersen, M.B.; Brannstrom, M. Mayer-Rokitansky-Kuster-Hauser (MRKH) syndrome: A comprehensive update. *Orphanet. J. Rare. Dis.* **2020**, *15*, 214. [CrossRef] [PubMed]
2. Rall, K.; Eisenbeis, S.; Henninger, V.; Henes, M.; Wallwiener, D.; Bonin, M.; Brucker, S. Typical and Atypical Associated Findings in a Group of 346 Patients with Mayer-Rokitansky-Kuester-Hauser Syndrome. *J. Pediatr. Adolesc. Gynecol.* **2015**, *28*, 362–368. [CrossRef] [PubMed]
3. Blontzos, N.; Iavazzo, C.; Vorgias, G.; Kalinoglou, N. Leiomyoma development in Mayer-Rokitansky-Kuster-Hauser syndrome: A case report and a narrative review of the literature. *Obstet. Gynecol. Sci.* **2019**, *62*, 294–297. [CrossRef] [PubMed]
4. Romano, F.; Carlucci, S.; Stabile, G.; Mirenda, G.; Mirandola, M.; Mangino, F.P.; Romano, A.; Ricci, G. The Rare, Unexpected Condition of a Twisted Leiomyoma in Mayer-Rokitansky-Kuster-Hauser (MRKH) Syndrome: Etiopathogenesis, Diagnosis and Management. Our Experience and Narrative Review of the Literature. *Int. J. Environ. Res. Public. Health* **2021**, *18*, 5895. [CrossRef]

5. Chmel, R., Jr.; Novackova, M.; Chubanovova, N.; Pastor, Z. Sexuality in women with Mayer-Rokitansky-Kuster-Hauser syndrome. *Ceska Gynekol.* **2021**, *86*, 194–199. [CrossRef]
6. Herlin, M.; Hojland, A.T.; Petersen, M.B. Familial occurrence of Mayer-Rokitansky-Kuster-Hauser syndrome: A case report and review of the literature. *Am. J. Med. Genet. A* **2014**, *164*, 2276–2286. [CrossRef]
7. Chen, N.; Zhao, S.; Jolly, A.; Wang, L.; Pan, H.; Yuan, J.; Chen, S.; Koch, A.; Ma, C.; Tian, W.; et al. Perturbations of genes essential for Mullerian duct and Wolffian duct development in Mayer-Rokitansky-Kuster-Hauser syndrome. *Am. J. Hum. Genet.* **2021**, *108*, 337–345. [CrossRef]
8. Mikhael, S.; Dugar, S.; Morton, M.; Chorich, L.P.; Tam, K.B.; Lossie, A.C.; Kim, H.G.; Knight, J.; Taylor, H.S.; Mukherjee, S.; et al. Genetics of agenesis/hypoplasia of the uterus and vagina: Narrowing down the number of candidate genes for Mayer-Rokitansky-Kuster-Hauser Syndrome. *Hum. Genet.* **2021**, *140*, 667–680. [CrossRef]
9. Kyei Barffour, I.; Kyei Baah Kwarkoh, R. GREB1L as a candidate gene of Mayer-Rokitansky-Kuster-Hauser Syndrome. *Eur. J. Med. Genet.* **2021**, *64*, 104158. [CrossRef]
10. Backhouse, B.; Hanna, C.; Robevska, G.; van den Bergen, J.; Pelosi, E.; Simons, C.; Koopman, P.; Juniarto, A.Z.; Grover, S.; Faradz, S.; et al. Identification of Candidate Genes for Mayer-Rokitansky-Kuster-Hauser Syndrome Using Genomic Approaches. *Sex Dev.* **2019**, *13*, 26–34. [CrossRef]
11. Ledig, S.; Wieacker, P. Clinical and genetic aspects of Mayer-Rokitansky-Kuster-Hauser syndrome. *Med. Genet.* **2018**, *30*, 3–11. [CrossRef] [PubMed]
12. Pan, H.X.; Luo, G.N.; Wan, S.Q.; Qin, C.L.; Tang, J.; Zhang, M.; Du, M.; Xu, K.K.; Shi, J.Q. Detection of de novo genetic variants in Mayer-Rokitansky-Kuster-Hauser syndrome by whole genome sequencing. *Eur. J. Obstet. Gynecol. Reprod. Biol. X* **2019**, *4*, 100089. [CrossRef] [PubMed]
13. Lischke, J.H.; Curtis, C.H.; Lamb, E.J. Discordance of vaginal agenesis in monozygotic twins. *Obstet. Gynecol.* **1973**, *41*, 920–924. [PubMed]
14. Regenstein, A.C.; Berkeley, A.S. Discordance of mullerian agenesis in monozygotic twins. A case report. *J. Reprod. Med.* **1991**, *36*, 396–397.
15. Steinkam800f, M.P.; Dharia, S.P.; Dickerson, R.D. Monozygotic twins discordant for vaginal agenesis and bilateral tibial longitudinal deficiency. *Fertil. Steril.* **2003**, *80*, 643–645. [CrossRef]
16. Hentrich, T.; Koch, A.; Weber, N.; Kilzheimer, A.; Maia, A.; Burkhardt, S.; Rall, K.; Casadei, N.; Kohlbacher, O.; Riess, O.; et al. The Endometrial Transcription Landscape of MRKH Syndrome. *Front. Cell. Dev. Biol.* **2020**, *8*, 572281. [CrossRef]
17. Andrews, S. FastQC: A quality control tool for high throughput sequence data. 2010, in press. Available online: http://www.bioinformatics.babraham.ac.uk/projects/fastqc (accessed on 15 June 2021).
18. Dobin, A.; Davis, C.A.; Schlesinger, F.; Drenkow, J.; Zaleski, C.; Jha, S.; Batut, P.; Chaisson, M.; Gingeras, T.R. STAR: Ultrafast universal RNA-seq aligner. *Bioinformatics* **2013**, *29*, 15–21. [CrossRef]
19. Li, H.; Handsaker, B.; Wysoker, A.; Fennell, T.; Ruan, J.; Homer, N.; Marth, G.; Abecasis, G.; Durbin, R.; Genome Project Data Processing Subgroup. The Sequence Alignment/Map format and SAMtools. *Bioinformatics* **2009**, *25*, 2078–2079. [CrossRef]
20. Love, M.I.; Huber, W.; Anders, S. Moderated estimation of fold change and dispersion for RNA-seq data with DESeq2. *Genome Biol.* **2014**, *15*, 550. [CrossRef]
21. Srinivasan, K.; Friedman, B.A.; Larson, J.L.; Lauffer, B.E.; Goldstein, L.D.; Appling, L.L.; Borneo, J.; Poon, C.; Ho, T.; Cai, F.; et al. Untangling the brain's neuroinflammatory and neurodegenerative transcriptional responses. *Nat. Commun.* **2016**, *7*, 11295. [CrossRef]
22. Shannon, P.; Markiel, A.; Ozier, O.; Baliga, N.S.; Wang, J.T.; Ramage, D.; Amin, N.; Schwikowski, B.; Ideker, T. Cytoscape: A software environment for integrated models of biomolecular interaction networks. *Genome Res.* **2003**, *13*, 2498–2504. [CrossRef] [PubMed]
23. Wang, W.; Vilella, F.; Alama, P.; Moreno, I.; Mignardi, M.; Isakova, A.; Pan, W.; Simon, C.; Quake, S.R. Single-cell transcriptomic atlas of the human endometrium during the menstrual cycle. *Nat. Med.* **2020**, *26*, 1644–1653. [CrossRef] [PubMed]
24. De Tomasi, L.; David, P.; Humbert, C.; Silbermann, F.; Arrondel, C.; Tores, F.; Fouquet, S.; Desgrange, A.; Niel, O.; Bole-Feysot, C.; et al. Mutations in GREB1L Cause Bilateral Kidney Agenesis in Humans and Mice. *Am. J. Hum. Genet.* **2017**, *101*, 803–814. [CrossRef]
25. Schrauwen, I.; Liaqat, K.; Schatteman, I.; Bharadwaj, T.; Nasir, A.; Acharya, A.; Ahmad, W.; Van Camp, G.; Leal, S.M. Autosomal Dominantly Inherited GREB1L Variants in Individuals with Profound Sensorineural Hearing Impairment. *Genes* **2020**, *11*, 687. [CrossRef]
26. Wang, M.; Li, Y.; Ma, W.; Li, H.; He, F.; Pu, D.; Su, T.; Wang, S. Analysis of WNT9B mutations in Chinese women with Mayer-Rokitansky-Kuster-Hauser syndrome. *Reprod. Biomed. Online* **2014**, *28*, 80–85. [CrossRef] [PubMed]
27. Waschk, D.E.; Tewes, A.C.; Romer, T.; Hucke, J.; Kapczuk, K.; Schippert, C.; Hillemanns, P.; Wieacker, P.; Ledig, S. Mutations in WNT9B are associated with Mayer-Rokitansky-Kuster-Hauser syndrome. *Clin. Genet.* **2016**, *89*, 590–596. [CrossRef]
28. Karczewski, K.J.; Francioli, L.C.; Tiao, G.; Cummings, B.B.; Alfoldi, J.; Wang, Q.; Collins, R.L.; Laricchia, K.M.; Ganna, A.; Birnbaum, D.P.; et al. The mutational constraint spectrum quantified from variation in 141,456 humans. *Nature* **2020**, *581*, 434–443. [CrossRef]
29. Carlson, R.W. The history and mechanism of action of fulvestrant. *Clin. Breast. Cancer* **2005**, *6*, S5–S8. [CrossRef]
30. Nathan, M.R.; Schmid, P. A Review of Fulvestrant in Breast Cancer. *Oncol. Ther.* **2017**, *5*, 17–29. [CrossRef]

31. Kyei-Barffour, I.; Margetts, M.; Vash-Margita, A.; Pelosi, E. The Embryological Landscape of Mayer-Rokitansky-Kuster-Hauser Syndrome: Genetics and Environmental Factors. *Yale J. Biol. Med.* **2021**, *94*, 657–672.
32. Jonsson, H.; Magnusdottir, E.; Eggertsson, H.P.; Stefansson, O.A.; Arnadottir, G.A.; Eiriksson, O.; Zink, F.; Helgason, E.A.; Jonsdottir, I.; Gylfason, A.; et al. Differences between germline genomes of monozygotic twins. *Nat. Genet.* **2021**, *53*, 27–34. [CrossRef] [PubMed]
33. Rall, K.; Eisenbeis, S.; Barresi, G.; Ruckner, D.; Walter, M.; Poths, S.; Wallwiener, D.; Riess, O.; Bonin, M.; Brucker, S. Mayer-Rokitansky-Kuster-Hauser syndrome discordance in monozygotic twins: Matrix metalloproteinase 14, low-density lipoprotein receptor-related protein 10, extracellular matrix, and neoangiogenesis genes identified as candidate genes in a tissue-specific mosaicism. *Fertil. Steril.* **2015**, *103*, 494–502 e493.
34. Ringwald, M.; Baldock, R.; Bard, J.; Kaufman, M.; Eppig, J.T.; Richardson, J.E.; Nadeau, J.H.; Davidson, D. A database for mouse development. *Science* **1994**, *265*, 2033–2034. [CrossRef] [PubMed]
35. Brophy, P.D.; Rasmussen, M.; Parida, M.; Bonde, G.; Darbro, B.W.; Hong, X.; Clarke, J.C.; Peterson, K.A.; Denegre, J.; Schneider, M.; et al. A Gene Implicated in Activation of Retinoic Acid Receptor Targets Is a Novel Renal Agenesis Gene in Humans. *Genetics* **2017**, *207*, 215–228. [CrossRef] [PubMed]
36. Herlin, M.K.; Le, V.Q.; Hojland, A.T.; Ernst, A.; Okkels, H.; Petersen, A.C.; Petersen, M.B.; Pedersen, I.S. Whole-exome sequencing identifies a GREB1L variant in a three-generation family with Mullerian and renal agenesis: A novel candidate gene in Mayer-Rokitansky-Kuster-Hauser (MRKH) syndrome. A case report. *Hum. Reprod.* **2019**, *34*, 1838–1846. [CrossRef]
37. Sanna-Cherchi, S.; Khan, K.; Westland, R.; Krithivasan, P.; Fievet, L.; Rasouly, H.M.; Ionita-Laza, I.; Capone, V.P.; Fasel, D.A.; Kiryluk, K.; et al. Exome-wide Association Study Identifies GREB1L Mutations in Congenital Kidney Malformations. *Am. J. Hum. Genet.* **2017**, *101*, 789–802. [CrossRef]
38. Carroll, T.J.; Park, J.S.; Hayashi, S.; Majumdar, A.; McMahon, A.P. Wnt9b plays a central role in the regulation of mesenchymal to epithelial transitions underlying organogenesis of the mammalian urogenital system. *Dev. Cell* **2005**, *9*, 283–292. [CrossRef]
39. Kobayashi, A.; Behringer, R.R. Developmental genetics of the female reproductive tract in mammals. *Nat. Rev. Genet.* **2003**, *4*, 969–980. [CrossRef]
40. Ma, Y.; Li, Y.; Wang, M.; Li, H.; Su, T.; Li, Y.; Wang, S. Associations of Polymorphisms in WNT9B and PBX1 with Mayer-Rokitansky-Kuster-Hauser Syndrome in Chinese Han. *PLoS ONE* **2015**, *10*, e0130202. [CrossRef]
41. Tang, R.; Dang, Y.; Qin, Y.; Zou, S.; Li, G.; Wang, Y.; Chen, Z.J. WNT9B in 542 Chinese women with Mullerian duct abnormalities: Mutation analysis. *Reprod. Biomed. Online* **2014**, *28*, 503–507. [CrossRef]
42. Mansouri, A.; Chowdhury, K.; Gruss, P. Follicular cells of the thyroid gland require Pax8 gene function. *Nat. Genet.* **1998**, *19*, 87–90. [CrossRef]
43. Bouchard, M.; Pfeffer, P.; Busslinger, M. Functional equivalence of the transcription factors Pax2 and Pax5 in mouse development. *Development* **2000**, *127*, 3703–3713. [CrossRef]
44. Torres, M.; Gomez-Pardo, E.; Dressler, G.R.; Gruss, P. Pax-2 controls multiple steps of urogenital development. *Development* **1995**, *121*, 4057–4065. [CrossRef]
45. Mittag, J.; Winterhager, E.; Bauer, K.; Grummer, R. Congenital hypothyroid female pax8-deficient mice are infertile despite thyroid hormone replacement therapy. *Endocrinology* **2007**, *148*, 719–725. [CrossRef]
46. Smol, T.; Ribero-Karrouz, W.; Edery, P.; Gorduza, D.B.; Catteau-Jonard, S.; Manouvrier-Hanu, S.; Ghoumid, J. Mayer-Rokitansky-Kunster-Hauser syndrome due to 2q12.1q14.1 deletion: PAX8 the causing gene? *Eur. J. Med. Genet.* **2020**, *63*, 103812. [CrossRef]
47. Brucker, S.Y.; Eisenbeis, S.; Konig, J.; Lamy, M.; Salker, M.S.; Zeng, N.; Seeger, H.; Henes, M.; Scholler, D.; Schonfisch, B.; et al. Decidualization is Impaired in Endometrial Stromal Cells from Uterine Rudiments in Mayer-Rokitansky-Kuster-Hauser Syndrome. *Cell Physiol. Biochem.* **2017**, *41*, 1083–1097. [CrossRef]
48. Brucker, S.Y.; Frank, L.; Eisenbeis, S.; Henes, M.; Wallwiener, D.; Riess, O.; van Eijck, B.; Scholler, D.; Bonin, M.; Rall, K.K. Sequence variants in ESR1 and OXTR are associated with Mayer-Rokitansky-Kuster-Hauser syndrome. *Acta. Obstet. Gynecol. Scand.* **2017**, *96*, 1338–1346. [CrossRef]
49. Rall, K.; Barresi, G.; Walter, M.; Poths, S.; Haebig, K.; Schaeferhoff, K.; Schoenfisch, B.; Riess, O.; Wallwiener, D.; Bonin, M.; et al. A combination of transcriptome and methylation analyses reveals embryologically-relevant candidate genes in MRKH patients. *Orphanet. J. Rare Dis.* **2011**, *6*, 32. [CrossRef]
50. Masse, J.; Watrin, T.; Laurent, A.; Deschamps, S.; Guerrier, D.; Pellerin, I. The developing female genital tract: From genetics to epigenetics. *Int. J. Dev. Biol.* **2009**, *53*, 411–424. [CrossRef]
51. Block, K.; Kardana, A.; Igarashi, P.; Taylor, H.S. In utero diethylstilbestrol (DES) exposure alters Hox gene expression in the developing mullerian system. *FASEB J.* **2000**, *14*, 1101–1108. [CrossRef]
52. Kaufman, R.H.; Adam, E.; Hatch, E.E.; Noller, K.; Herbst, A.L.; Palmer, J.R.; Hoover, R.N. Continued follow-up of pregnancy outcomes in diethylstilbestrol-exposed offspring. *Obstet. Gynecol.* **2000**, *96*, 483–489. [PubMed]
53. Wautier, A.; Tournaire, M.; Devouche, E.; Epelboin, S.; Pouly, J.L.; Levadou, A. Genital tract and reproductive characteristics in daughters of women and men prenatally exposed to diethylstilbestrol (DES). *Therapie* **2020**, *75*, 439–448. [CrossRef] [PubMed]
54. Petrozza, J.C.; Gray, M.R.; Davis, A.J.; Reindollar, R.H. Congenital absence of the uterus and vagina is not commonly transmitted as a dominant genetic trait: Outcomes of surrogate pregnancies. *Fertil. Steril.* **1997**, *67*, 387–389. [CrossRef]
55. Albers, C.A.; Newbury-Ecob, R.; Ouwehand, W.H.; Ghevaert, C. New insights into the genetic basis of TAR (thrombocytopenia-absent radii) syndrome. *Curr. Opin. Genet. Dev.* **2013**, *23*, 316–323. [CrossRef]

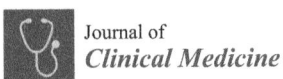

Article

Endometriosis in Patients with Mayer-Rokitansky-Küster-Hauser-Syndrome—Histological Evaluation of Uterus Remnants and Peritoneal Lesions and Comparison to Samples from Endometriosis Patients without Mullerian Anomaly

Sahra Steinmacher [1,*], Hans Bösmüller [2], Massimo Granai [2], André Koch [1], Sara Yvonne Brucker [1] and Kristin Katharina Rall [1]

1. Department of Women's Health, Tuebingen University Hospital, Calwerstr 7, 72076 Tuebingen, Germany
2. Department of Pathology, Tuebingen University Hospital, Liebermeisterstraße 8, 72076 Tuebingen, Germany
* Correspondence: sahra.steinmacher@med.uni-tuebingen.de; Tel.: +49-7071-29-82211

Abstract: Congenital Mayer-Rokitansky-Küster-Hauser (MRKH) syndrome is a Mullerian-duct anomaly that is characterized by agenesis of the uterus and upper part of the vagina. Uterus remnants of varying sizes can often be found. Although a functional uterus is missing, the existence of endometriosis in this patient group has been described in the literature; however, a histopathological comparison of the characteristics of the endometrium within the uterus remnants versus endometriotic peritoneal lesions in the same patient is lacking. Moreover, the characteristics of endometriotic tissue in patients with MRKH syndrome have not been correlated with those of patients with endometriosis without Mullerian anomaly. Patients who underwent laparoscopic neovagina creation with the removal of uterus remnants and possible resection of endometriotic lesions between 2010 and 2022 at the Department of Women's health of the University of Tuebingen were included in our study. Uterine remnants and endometriotic tissue were evaluated via histopathology and immunohistochemistry and were compared to endometriotic samples from patients without Mullerian anomaly. Endometriosis was detected in nine MRKH patients; in four patients, endometrial remnants could be sufficiently compared to endometriotic lesions. All samples exhibited increased expression of hormonal receptors. In two patients, Ki67 proliferation index was significantly increased in peritoneal endometriotic lesions compared with the endometrium of the remnants. In contrast, endometrium and endometriotic lesions of endometriosis patients did not exhibit any differences in the Ki67 proliferation index. Our results demonstrate distinctive immunohistochemical variability between uterine remnants and endometriotic lesions in patients with MRKH syndrome compared with patients with endometriosis, indicating a possible explanation model of the yet-unknown etiology of endometriosis. For confirmation, investigation of a broader patient collective is necessary.

Keywords: Mayer-Rokitansky-Küster-Hauser syndrome; endometriosis; uterus remnants; uterus aplasia

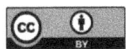

1. Introduction

Congenital MRKH syndrome is a Mullerian duct anomaly that is characterized by agenesis of the uterus and upper part of the vagina with normal secondary sex characteristics and normal female karyotype. It is the second most common cause of primary amenorrhea after gonadal dysgenesis and occurs in about 1 of 4500 female live births [1–3]. MRKH syndrome is classified as type 1, where an isolated uterovaginal aplasia can be diagnosed, or type 2 with associated extragenital malformations [4].

Uterine remnants can be seen in from 50% to almost 100% of all MRKH patients [5–7], whereas the endometrium can be histologically detected in up to 50% of all surgically removed remnants [5,8]. About one-half of these patients experience recurrent cyclic symptoms caused by proliferation of the endometrium, endometriosis, or myomas [8–11].

Endometriosis is defined as the existence of endometrial glands and stroma in extrauterine locations. It is an estrogen-dependent, inflammatory condition associated with pelvic pain and infertility [12].

To date a unifying theory of the origin of endometriosis is lacking. Generally theories can be classified as those promoting that endometriotic implants originate from uterine endometrium, whereas others state that implants originate from tissues other than the uterus [12]. MRKH syndrome with uterine remnants and functional endometrium is a rare subtype within the obstructive Mullerian duct anomalies. The etiology of MRKH syndrome is currently unknown. In a study by Brucker et al., endometrial stroma cells derived from patients with MRKH syndrome exhibited significantly less decidualization compared with healthy controls in addition to lower hormone responsiveness, possibly indicating a dysfunctional hormone receptor function that may play a role in the etiology of MRKH syndrome [13]. Furthermore, uterine remnants in patients with MRKH syndrome were found to contain typical uterine tissue with a more basalis-like endometrium and significantly lower proliferation compared with healthy controls [5].

Various studies have demonstrated the occurrence of endometriosis in patients with MRKH syndrome [14,15] and its clinical features [16].

To date, the histological features of endometriosis in patients with MRKH syndrome in comparison with healthy patients have not been elucidated.

We sought to analyze possible differences between the endometrium in uterine remnants and endometriotic lesions in patients with MRKH syndrome compared to samples from patients with endometriosis, to achieve new insights into the etiology and pathogenesis of MRKH syndrome and, possibly, endometriosis.

2. Material and Methods

Our study was a retrospective histological analysis of endometriotic tissue and endometrium of uterine remnants from patients with MRKH syndrome and their comparison to samples from patients with endometriosis. Tissue was obtained from patients with MRKH after informed consent. Patients underwent laparoscopically assisted creation of a neovagina using the modified Vecchietti technique (described elsewhere) at the Department of Obstetrics and Gynecology of the University of Tuebingen between 2010 and 2022 [17,18]. Patients with endometriosis simultaneously received a hysterectomy and removal of endometriotic tissue.

Correlation with the individual cycle phase was performed by obtaining standardized medical history and using hormone profiles from peripheral blood taken 1 day before surgery.

Every patient underwent a preoperative uro-MRI to exclude anomalies of the urogenital tract.

The study was approved by the Ethics Committee of Eberhard-Karls-University of Tuebingen (205/2014BO1).

2.1. Histologic Analysis

Endometriotic lesions and corresponding endometrial tissue were evaluated by an experienced gynecological pathologist. Macroscopic description was performed, and the sample was cut perpendicular to the longest axis. One section was cryopreserved, and the remaining specimen was fixed in formalin and embedded in paraffin. Sections of 2.5 µm were cut from each block and stained with hematoxylin and eosin (H & E).

2.2. Immunohistochemistry

Immunohistochemistry was performed using Ventana Discovery automated immunostaining system and Ventana reagents (Ventana Medical Systems). We took 2.5 µm-Sections from the respective specimen blocks and mounted them on Superfrost slides (Langenbrinck, Bern, Switzerland). Sections were deparaffinized with inorganic buffer. Pretreatment with ethylenediaminetetraacetic acid (EDTA) buffer was performed. EDTA-buffer was used pH 8.0 for estrogen receptor (ER), pH 6.0 for progesterone receptor (PR) and pH 8.4 for Ki67. Heat-induced epitope retrieval was performed for every antigen. Then, the primary antibody was applied for 1 h at room temperature (monoclonal rabbit anti-human ER, cone SP1, (DCS innovative Diagnostik Systeme, Hamburg, Germany); dilution 1:100, antibody diluent (Zytomed Systems, Berlin, Germany); monoclonal rabbit anti-human PR, clone SP2, (DCS innovative Diagnostik Systeme, Hamburg, Germany), dilution 1:150, antibody diluent DCS diluent; monoclonal mouse anti-human Ki-67-Antigen, clone MiB-1, M7240, (DakoCytomation, Glostrup, Denmark), dilution 1:400, antibody diluent Zytomed Systems, Berlin, Germany). A biotinylated detection kit including diaminobenzidine and horseradish peroxidase (DABMap Kit Ventana, Roche, Rotkreuz, Switzerland) was utilized. Counterstaining with hematoxylin and Blueing Reagent (Roche 760-2021) was performed. Slides were then washed and dehydrated with a series of ascending alcohol concentrations (40%, 70%, 96%) and covered with Cytoseal (Thermo Scientific, Waltham, MA, USA).

Nonexpressing tissues and staining protocols without the primary antibody were used as internal negative control.

2.3. Interpretation of Immunostaining Results

2.3.1. Estrogen and Progesterone Receptor

ER and PR were quantified with the scoring system according to Remmele and Stegner [19]. The intensity of the nuclear stain was scored from 0 to 3 and then multiplied with a score for the number of positive cells (score 0 = 0, score 1 = 1–10%, score 2 = 11–50%, score 3 = 51–80%, score 4 = 81–100%), producing a score from 0 to 12.

2.3.2. MiB1 (Antibody against Ki67)

The percentage of positive nuclei was estimated by evaluation of at least 100 cells in one distinct area in the respective compartment of the specimen.

2.4. Hormone Profile and Correlation with Cycle Phase

Whole blood collection from patients with MRKH and endometriosis was performed 1 day before or after surgery. Estrogen, progesterone, luteinizing hormone (LH) and follicle-stimulating hormone (FSH) was measured in blood serum using a chemiluminescence immunoassay (Vitros eci, Madrid, Spain; Diagnostic Product Coorperation).

The proliferative phase (cycle phase 1) was assigned when progesterone was <2.5 ng/mL, and the secretory phase (cycle phase 2) when progesterone was >5 ng/mL and the LH/FSH ratio was >1.5.

3. Results

Of the 319 patients who underwent neovagina creation between 2010 and 2021 and the additional removal of uterine remnants, endometriotic tissue was detected in 9 patients (3.1%).

Median age of patients at time of surgery was 23.5 years (IQR 18.25–32).

Adenomyosis was diagnosed within the uterine remnants in five patients; adenomyosis and endometriotic peritoneal lesions were found in one patient; one patient was diagnosed with endometriosis in the peritoneum, ovary and remnants; endometriosis was detected in the ovaries in two patients.

None of the patients had associated malformations. Three patients reported cyclic abdominal pain.

Uterine remnants were located bilaterally in all patients. One patient had previously undergone removal of remnants. Hematometra due to endometrial proliferation was not diagnosed in any of the patients. In one patient with a severe endometriosis and prominent remnants, the fallopian tubes were altered similarly to a hemato- or sactosalpinx.

The cycle phase was evaluated by obtaining a hormonal profile from peripheral blood taken 1 day before or after surgery. Six patients were in cycle phase 1 (proliferative phase), one patient was in cycle phase 2 (secretory phase), and the cycle phase was unknown in three patients (for details see Table 1).

Table 1. Clinical characteristics.

Patient Number	Age at Surgery	Existing Uterus Remnants	Adenomyosis	Localization of Endometriosis	Clinical Symptoms	Associated Malformations	Hormonal Profile
1	16	Both sides	No	Right ovary	Abdominal pain	None	N/A
1	23	Removed	/	Right ovary	Unknown	None	N/A
2	49	Both sides	Yes	Adenomyosis	None	None	N/A
3	16	Both sides	No	Peritoneum	None	None	Cycle phase 1
4	19	Both sides	Yes (left side)	Adenomyosis	None	None	Cycle phase 2/periovulatory
5	24	Both sides	Yes	Peritoneum	Cyclic abdominal pain	None	Cycle phase 1
6	27	Both sides	Yes (left side)	Adenomyosis	None	None	Cycle phase 1
7	29	Both sides	Yes (right side)	Adenomyosis	Unknown	None	Cycle phase 1
8	20	Both sides	Yes (left side)	Adenomyosis	Cyclic abdominal pain	None	Cycle phase 1
9	41	Both sides	Yes (both sides)	Peritoneum	None	None	Cycle phase 1

N/A, not available.

The expression of hormonal receptors was evaluated in the uterine remnants of five patients, as endometrial specimens from the remaining patients were too small for immunohistochemistry. All specimens exhibited a high expression of estrogen and progesterone receptor (IRS 12). In the corresponding endometriotic lesions, expression of hormonal receptors was more heterogeneous. The expression of progesterone receptor was lower in epithelial cells than in stromal cells in the two ovarian endometriotic specimens. In two patients, estrogen-receptor expression in the endometriotic tissue was comparably lower than in the corresponding uterine remnants.

The proliferation marker Ki67 differed significantly in two patients when comparing the proliferation in the endometriotic tissue to the remnants, as Mib was significantly lower in the remnants than in the endometriotic specimens ($p = 0.0254$). Both patients were in the proliferative phase. In two patients, Ki67 was <1% in both the endometriotic tissue and uterine remnants (for details, see Table 2).

Endometriotic tissue and the corresponding endometrium were analyzed in two patients with endometriosis. The two patients were 37 and 39 years old and both were premenopausal. They did not take any hormonal therapy. One patient presented with endometriosis of the bladder and subsequent partial removal of the bladder during surgery. The other patient had extensive peritoneal endometriosis (rASRM stage 4). One patient was in the proliferative and one in the secretory cycle phase at the timepoint of surgery. Both the endometrial and the endometriotic tissue of the patient in the proliferative phase exhibited increased expression of the estrogen-receptor (IRS 12). Ki67 was 40% both in the endometrial and in endometriotic tissue. Samples from the patient in the secretory phase demonstrated a heterogenous moderate-to-strong expression of the estrogen-receptor in 75% of the epithelium, in both endometrial and endometriotic tissue. Ki67 was 0% in both the endometriotic and endometrial tissue (for details, see Figures 1–7).

Table 2. Results for immunohistochemistry IRS (ER, PR) and Ki67.

Patient Number	Estrogen Receptor Expression Uterus Remnants	Progesterone Receptor Expression Uterus Remnants	Estrogen Receptor Expression Endometriotic Lesion	Progesterone Receptor Expression Endometriotic Lesion	Ki67 Uterus Remnants	Ki67 Endometriotic Lesion
1	12	12	6	4 (stroma 12)	<1%	<1%
1	N/A	N/A	9	4 (stroma 12)	N/A	8%
2	12	9	N/A	N/A	N/A	N/A
3	12	12	4	12	15%	75%
4	12	12	N/A	N/A	5%	N/A
5	N/A	N/A	N/A	N/A	N/A	N/A
6	N/A	N/A	N/A	N/A	N/A	N/A
7	N/A	N/A	N/A	N/A	N/A	N/A
8	12	12	12	9	<1%	1%
9	12	12	12	12	15%	80%

N/A, not available.

Comparison of uterus remnant and endometriotic specimen in a patient with MRKH (Figures 1–3).

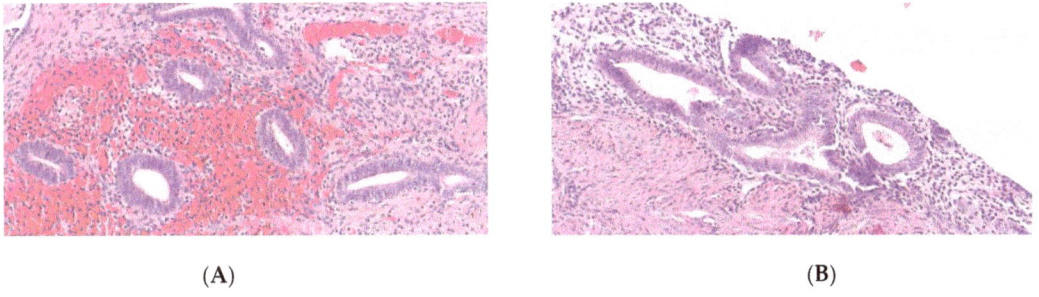

(A)   (B)

Figure 1. Hematoxylin and eosin (H&E) staining (×200). (A) endometriosis. (B) uterus remnant.

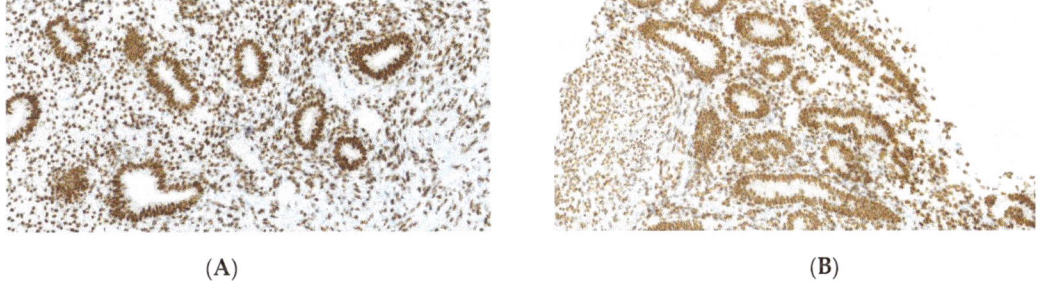

(A)   (B)

Figure 2. Estrogen receptor (ER) with strong nuclear expression (×200). (A) endometriosis. (B) uterus remnant.

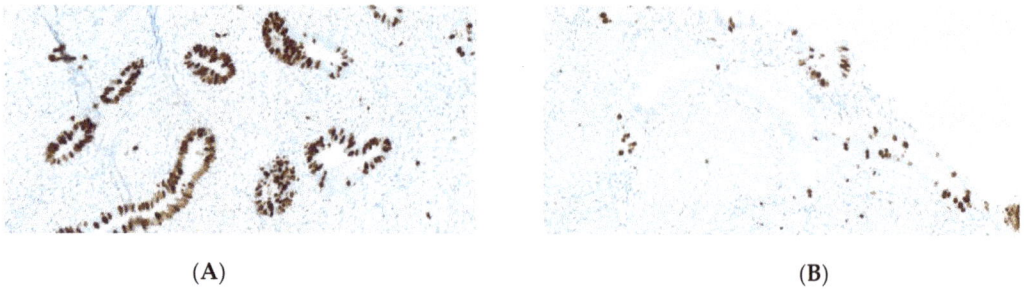

Figure 3. Immunohistochemistry for K67 (MiB1), demonstrating higher proliferative index in endometriosis than in the uterine remnant (×200). (**A**) endometriosis. (**B**) uterus remnant.

Comparison of uterine endometrium and endometriotic specimen in healthy patients. Patient in proliferative phase (Figures 4–6).

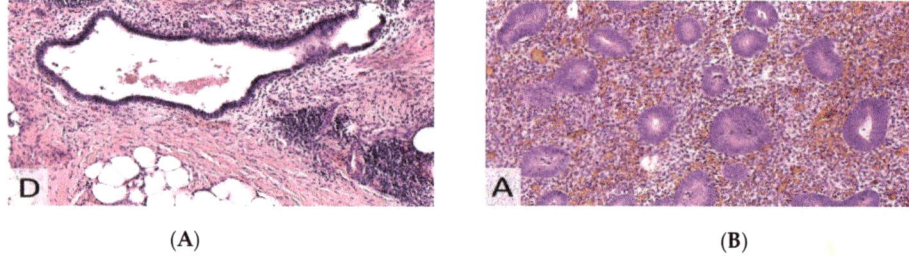

Figure 4. Hematoxylin and eosin (H&E) staining (×200). (**A**) Endometriosis. (**B**) Endometrium.

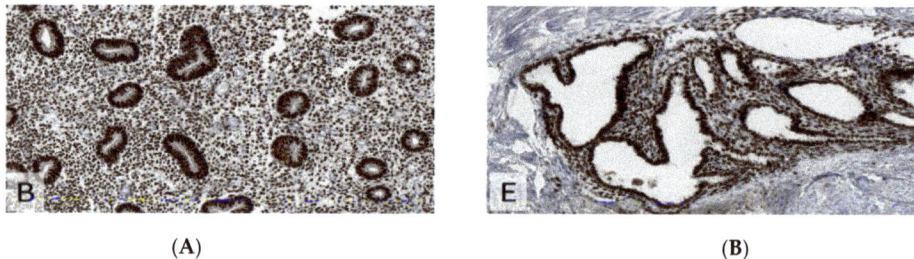

Figure 5. Estrogen receptor (ER) with strong nuclear expression (IRS 12) (×200). (**A**) Endometriosis. (**B**) Endometrium.

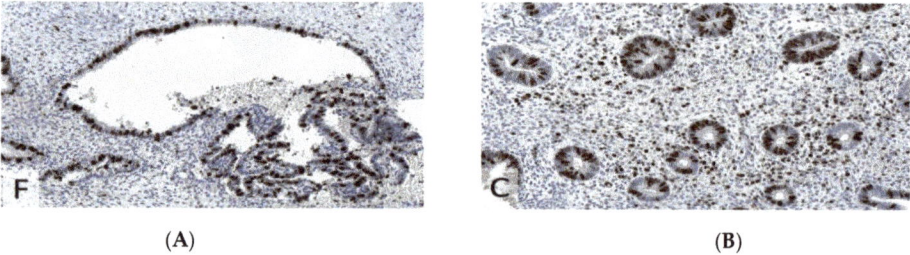

Figure 6. IHC for Ki67 (MiB1), demonstrating the same proliferative index (40%) in endometriosis compared to endometrium (×200). (**A**) Endometriosis. (**B**) Endometrium.

Patient in secretory phase (Figures 7–9).

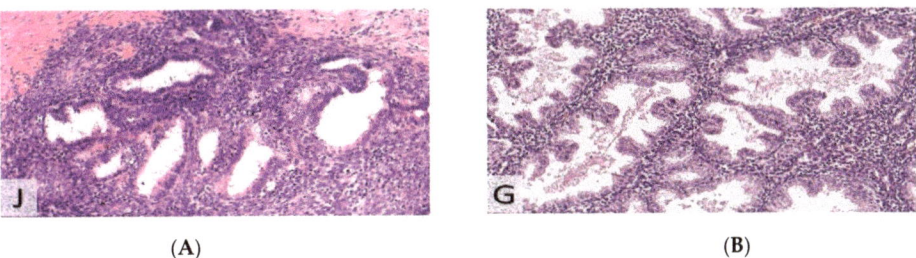

Figure 7. Hematoxylin and eosin (H&E) staining (×200). (**A**) Endometriosis. (**B**) Endometrium.

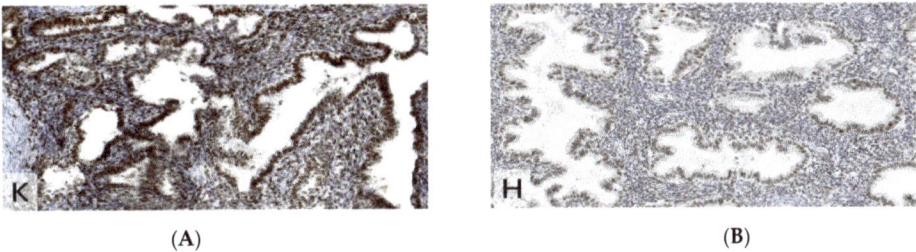

Figure 8. Estrogen receptor (ER) with heterogeneous moderate to strong expression in 75% of the epithelium (×200). (**A**) Endometriosis. (**B**) Endometrium.

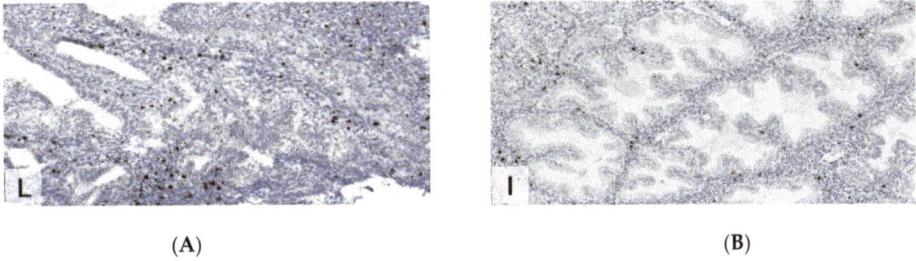

Figure 9. IHC for Ki67 (MiB1), demonstrating the same proliferative index (lower than in proliferative phase) in endometriosis compared to endometrium (×200). (**A**) Endometriosis. (**B**) Endometrium.

4. Discussion

To date, no study has investigated and compared the immunohistochemistry of uterine remnants and corresponding endometriotic lesions in MRKH patients with endometriotic samples of healthy patients. In our findings, there was no significant quantitative difference in the expression of hormonal receptors in endometriotic tissue and in the endometrium of uterine remnants in MRKH patients. Therefore, it remains unclear why the endometrium of the remnants was mostly dormant. This observation may possibly underline the hypothesis of deficient hormonal receptors in patients with MRKH syndrome [20].

Interestingly, in two patients with MRKH syndrome in our study, the Ki67 proliferation index was significantly higher in the peritoneal endometriotic lesion than in the uterine rudiments. This might suggest a differing origin of the endometriotic tissue compared to the uterine endometrium.

This is further underlined by the fact that, in contrast with the samples from MRKH patients, endometrial and endometriotic tissue from endometriosis patients did not exhibit any differences regarding immunohistochemical evaluation of the proliferation index and were concordant and adequate for the respective cycle phase.

Throughout history, obstructive Mullerian duct anomalies have served as an explanatory model to support the theory of retrograde menstruation, as an increased incidence of endometriosis was noted in patients with associated hematocolpos or hematometra [21].

Data on endometriosis in MRKH patients are mainly based on case reports; therefore, demographic data and incidence rates are sparse [8,14,22–29]. Considering the previous considerations, we assumed that the incidence of endometriosis in patients with MRKH syndrome and functioning endometrium would be at least as high as it was in the general population. Here, endometriosis is estimated to affect 10–15% of all women of reproductive age [30]. In contrast to general findings, the incidence of endometriosis in our patient collective was considerably lower.

In the aforementioned case reports, the authors reported mostly laparoscopically detected endometriomas, peritoneal lesions or adenomyosis; in some cases, the absence of functional endometrium in uterine remnants or a complete lack of uterine rudiments was reported.

These findings may emphasize the theory of coelomic metaplasia as a complementary factor in the development of endometriosis [31].

In contrast, Konrad et al. emphasized, in their review of endometriosis in MRKH patients, that many of these published case reports are missing evidence of the existence of uterine remnants, as diagnostics for uterine remnants are inconsistently based on MRI-diagnostics or two-dimensional ultrasound and rarely based on histological evidence [32]. Histological proof of endometriotic lesions was presented in only a few articles [22,25,26,31,33]. Konrad et al. highlighted that the existence of functional endometrial tissue in uterine remnants is essential for the development of endometriosis in MRKH patients. As endometriomas were the most common manifestation in these patients, the authors stated that coelomic metaplasia may have contributed to their development [32].

Therefore, the surgical removal of uterine remnants with functional endometrial tissue is recommended to minimize the risk of developing endometriosis or reduce its extent linked to retrograde menstruation [34].

In our study, six patients had histological proof of the existence of dormant endometrium in their rudiments, one patient presented with adenomyosis-like endometrial glands, and one patient had extensive prismatic epithelium within the remnant. Only one patient from our cohort, who was diagnosed with severe endometriosis, had proliferative endometrium in a uterine remnant. As all patients underwent blood collection for hormonal profiling at the time of surgery, it is surprising that almost all patients were in the first cycle phase; only one patient with dormant endometrium had a hormonal profile consistent with the second cycle phase.

The existence of endometrioma was reported in more than half of cases in the literature. Only two out of nine patients were diagnosed with endometrioma in our study. Diagnosis was made prior to surgery, as all patients received a preoperative MRI of the urogenital tract.

One limitation of our study is the small sample size. Due to the rarity of MRKH syndrome, it is challenging to establish a cohort with an adequate number of patients, even though our department can refer to the largest collective of patients with MRKH syndrome in Germany. Therefore, a future approach might be the implementation of international multi-center studies with standardized diagnostic criteria and histological evaluation to provide a larger patient cohort. Moreover, the comparison of endometriosis to more patients with endometriosis without Mullerian anomaly might produce relevant differences and potentially highlight new explanation models for the development of endometriosis, possibly promoting an extrauterine origin of the endometriotic implants.

5. Conclusions

Our results revealed significant immunohistochemical variability between uterine remnants and endometriotic lesions in patients with MRKH syndrome compared with samples from patients with endometriosis without Mullerian anomaly, indicating a possible explanation model for the yet-unknown etiology of endometriosis. Despite the increased expression of hormonal receptors in the endometrial tissue of remnants, the endometrium mainly remained dormant, even in the proliferative cycle phase, possibly underlining the hypothesis of deficient hormonal receptors in patients with MRKH syndrome. To confirm our findings, an international multi-center study with a standardized diagnostic procedure and sample collection is needed to estimate the true incidence of endometriosis in MRKH syndrome.

Author Contributions: Conceptualization, A.K. and K.K.R.; Data curation, S.S., H.B. and M.G.; Writing—original draft, S.S.; Writing—review & editing, H.B., M.G., A.K., S.Y.B. and K.K.R. All authors have read and agreed to the published version of the manuscript.

Funding: This research was funded by Open Access Publishing Fund of the University of Tübingen.

Institutional Review Board Statement: The study was conducted in accordance with the Declaration of Helsinki, and approved by the Institutional Review Board of Eberhard-Karls-University of Tuebingen (205/2014BO1).

Informed Consent Statement: Patient consent was waived due to rarity of the disease and public interest in the topic.

Data Availability Statement: The data presented in this study are available on request from the corresponding author. The data are not publicly available due to patient confidentiality.

Conflicts of Interest: The authors declare no conflict of interest.

References

1. Varner, R.E.; Younger, J.B.; Blackwell, R.E. Mullerian dysgenesis. *J. Reprod. Med.* **1985**, *30*, 443–450. [PubMed]
2. Aittomaki, K.; Eroila, H.; Kajanoja, P. A population-based study of the incidence of Mullerian aplasia in Finland. *Fertil. Steril.* **2001**, *76*, 624–625. [CrossRef]
3. Folch, M.; Pigem, I.; Konje, J.C. Mullerian agenesis: Etiology, diagnosis, and management. *Obstet. Gynecol. Surv.* **2000**, *55*, 644–649. [CrossRef]
4. Herlin, M.K.; Petersen, M.B.; Brannstrom, M. Mayer-Rokitansky-Kuster-Hauser (MRKH) syndrome: A comprehensive update. *Orphanet J. Rare Dis.* **2020**, *15*, 214. [CrossRef] [PubMed]
5. Rall, K.; Barresi, G.; Wallwiener, D.; Brucker, S.Y.; Staebler, A. Uterine rudiments in patients with Mayer-Rokitansky-Kuster-Hauser syndrome consist of typical uterine tissue types with predominantly basalis-like endometrium. *Fertil. Steril.* **2013**, *99*, 1392–1399. [CrossRef] [PubMed]
6. Oppelt, P.G.; Lermann, J.; Strick, R.; Dittrich, R.; Strissel, P.; Rettig, I.; Schulze, C.; Renner, S.P.; Beckmann, M.W.; Brucker, S.; et al. Malformations in a cohort of 284 women with Mayer-Rokitansky-Kuster-Hauser syndrome (MRKH). *Reprod. Biol. Endocrinol.* **2012**, *10*, 57. [CrossRef] [PubMed]
7. Preibsch, H.; Rall, K.; Wietek, B.M.; Brucker, S.Y.; Staebler, A.; Claussen, C.D.; Siegmann-Luz, K.C. Clinical value of magnetic resonance imaging in patients with Mayer-Rokitansky-Kuster-Hauser (MRKH) syndrome: Diagnosis of associated malformations, uterine rudiments and intrauterine endometrium. *Eur. Radiol.* **2014**, *24*, 1621–1627. [CrossRef]
8. Marsh, C.A.; Will, M.A.; Smorgick, N.; Quint, E.H.; Hussain, H.; Smith, Y.R. Uterine remnants and pelvic pain in females with Mayer-Rokitansky-Kuster-Hauser syndrome. *J. Pediatric Adolesc. Gynecol.* **2013**, *26*, 199–202. [CrossRef]
9. Fedele, L.; Bianchi, S.; Frontino, G.; Ciappina, N.; Fontana, E.; Borruto, F. Laparoscopic findings and pelvic anatomy in Mayer-Rokitansky-Kuster-Hauser syndrome. *Obstet. Gynecol.* **2007**, *109*, 1111–1115. [CrossRef]
10. Deligeoroglou, E.; Kontoravdis, A.; Makrakis, E.; Christopoulos, P.; Kountouris, A.; Creatsas, G. Development of leiomyomas on the uterine remnants of two women with Mayer-Rokitansky-Kuster-Hauser syndrome. *Fertil. Steril.* **2004**, *81*, 1385–1387. [CrossRef]
11. Papa, G.; Andreotti, M.; Giannubilo, S.R.; Cesari, R.; Cere, I.; Tranquilli, A.L. Case report and surgical solution for a voluminous uterine leiomyoma in a woman with complicated Mayer-Rokitansky-Kuster-Hauser syndrome. *Fertil. Steril.* **2008**, *90*, 2014.e5–2014.e6. [CrossRef]
12. Burney, R.O.; Giudice, L.C. Pathogenesis and pathophysiology of endometriosis. *Fertil. Steril.* **2012**, *98*, 511–519. [CrossRef] [PubMed]

13. Brucker, S.Y.; Eisenbeis, S.; König, J.; Lamy, M.; Salker, M.S.; Zeng, N.; Seeger, H.; Henes, M.; Schöller, D.; Schönfisch, B.; et al. Decidualization is Impaired in Endometrial Stromal Cells from Uterine Rudiments in Mayer-Rokitansky-Kuster-Hauser Syndrome. *Cell. Physiol. Biochem.* **2017**, *41*, 1083–1097. [CrossRef] [PubMed]
14. Mok-Lin, E.Y.; Wolfberg, A.; Hollinquist, H.; Laufer, M.R. Endometriosis in a patient with Mayer-Rokitansky-Kuster-Hauser syndrome and complete uterine agenesis: Evidence to support the theory of coelomic metaplasia. *J. Pediatr. Adolesc. Gynecol.* **2010**, *23*, e35–e37. [CrossRef] [PubMed]
15. Parkar, R.B.; Patel, Y. Laparoscopic management of uterine perforation: Report of three cases. *East Afr. Med. J.* **2009**, *86*, 143–145. [CrossRef]
16. Tian, W.; Chen, N.; Liang, Z.; Song, S.; Wang, Y.; Ye, Y.; Duan, J.; Zhu, L. Clinical Features and Management of Endometriosis among Patients with MRKH and Functional Uterine Remnants. *Gynecol. Obstet. Investig.* **2021**, *86*, 518–524. [CrossRef] [PubMed]
17. Brucker, S.Y.; Gegusch, M.; Zubke, W.; Rall, K.; Gauwerky, J.F.; Wallwiener, D. Neovagina creation in vaginal agenesis: Development of a new laparoscopic Vecchietti-based procedure and optimized instruments in a prospective comparative interventional study in 101 patients. *Fertil. Steril.* **2008**, *90*, 1940–1952. [CrossRef] [PubMed]
18. Rall, K.; Schickner, M.C.; Barresi, G.; Schonfisch, B.; Wallwiener, M.; Wallwiener, C.W.; Wallwiener, D.; Brucker, Y.S. Laparoscopically assisted neovaginoplasty in vaginal agenesis: A long-term outcome study in 240 patients. *J. Pediatr. Adolesc. Gynecol.* **2014**, *27*, 379–385. [CrossRef]
19. Remmele, W.; Stegner, H.E. Recommendation for uniform definition of an immunoreactive score (IRS) for immunohistochemical estrogen receptor detection (ER-ICA) in breast cancer tissue. *Pathologe* **1987**, *8*, 138–140.
20. Rall, K.; Barresi, G.; Walter, M.; Poths, S.; Haebig, K.; Schaeferhoff, K.; Schoenfisch, B.; Riess, O.; Wallwiener, D.; Bonin, M.; et al. A combination of transcriptome and methylation analyses reveals embryologically-relevant candidate genes in MRKH patients. *Orphanet J. Rare Dis.* **2011**, *6*, 32. [CrossRef]
21. Olive, D.L.; Henderson, D.Y. Endometriosis and mullerian anomalies. *Obstet. Gynecol.* **1987**, *69*, 412–415. [PubMed]
22. Cho, M.K.; Kim, C.H.; Oh, S.T. Endometriosis in a patient with Rokitansky-Kuster-Hauser syndrome. *J. Obstet. Gynaecol. Res.* **2009**, *35*, 994–996. [CrossRef] [PubMed]
23. Troncon, J.K.; Zani, A.C.; Vieira, A.D.; Poli-Neto, O.B.; Nogueira, A.A.; Rosa ESilva, J.C. Endometriosis in a patient with mayer-rokitansky-kuster-hauser syndrome. *Case Rep. Obstet. Gynecol.* **2014**, *2014*, 376231. [CrossRef] [PubMed]
24. Yan, C.M.; Mok, K.M. Uterine fibroids and adenomyosis in a woman with Rokitansky-Kuster-Hauser syndrome. *J. Obstet. Gynaecol.* **2002**, *22*, 561–562. [CrossRef]
25. Enatsu, A.; Harada, T.; Yoshida, S.; Iwabe, T.; Terakawa, N. Adenomyosis in a patient with the Rokitansky-Kuster-Hauser syndrome. *Fertil. Steril.* **2000**, *73*, 862–863. [CrossRef]
26. Kawano, Y.; Hirakawa, T.; Nishida, M.; Yuge, A.; Yano, M.; Nasu, K.; Narahara, H. Functioning endometrium and endometrioma in a patient with mayer-rokitanski-kuster-hauser syndrome. *Jpn. Clin. Med.* **2014**, *5*, 43–45. [CrossRef]
27. Acien, P.; Lloret, M.; Chehab, H. Endometriosis in a patient with Rokitansky-Kuster-Hauser syndrome. *Gynecol. Obstet. Invest.* **1988**, *25*, 70–72. [CrossRef]
28. Rosenfeld, D.L.; Lecher, B.D. Endometriosis in a patient with Rokitansky-Kuster-Hauser syndrome. *Am. J. Obstet. Gynecol.* **1981**, *139*, 105. [CrossRef]
29. Will, M.A.; Marsh, C.A.; Smorgick, N.; Smith, Y.R.; Quint, E.H. Surgical pearls: Laparoscopic removal of uterine remnants in patients with Mayer-Rokitansky-Kuster-Hauser syndrome. *J. Pediatr. Adolesc. Gynecol.* **2013**, *26*, 224–227. [CrossRef]
30. Taylor, H.S.; Kotlyar, A.M.; Flores, V.A. Endometriosis is a chronic systemic disease: Clinical challenges and novel innovations. *Lancet* **2021**, *397*, 839–852. [CrossRef]
31. Yan, L.; Zhao, X.; Qin, X. MRKH syndrome with endometriosis: Case report and literature review. *Eur. J. Obstet. Gynecol. Reprod. Biol.* **2011**, *159*, 231–232. [CrossRef] [PubMed]
32. Konrad, L.; Dietze, R.; Kudipudi, P.K.; Horne, F.; Meinhold-Heerlein, I. Endometriosis in MRKH cases as a proof for the coelomic metaplasia hypothesis? *Reproduction* **2019**, *158*, R41–R47. [CrossRef] [PubMed]
33. Chun, S.; Kim, Y.M.; Ji, Y.I. Uterine adenomyosis which developed from hypoplastic uterus in postmenopausal woman with mayer-rokitansky-kuster-hauser syndrome: A case report. *J. Menopausal. Med.* **2013**, *19*, 135–138. [CrossRef] [PubMed]
34. Committee on Adolescent Health Care. ACOG Committee Opinion No. 728: Mullerian Agenesis: Diagnosis, Management, and Treatment. *Obstet. Gynecol.* **2018**, *131*, e35–e42. [CrossRef] [PubMed]

MDPI
St. Alban-Anlage 66
4052 Basel
Switzerland
www.mdpi.com

Journal of Clinical Medicine Editorial Office
E-mail: jcm@mdpi.com
www.mdpi.com/journal/jcm

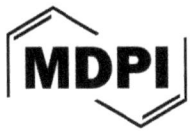

Disclaimer/Publisher's Note: The statements, opinions and data contained in all publications are solely those of the individual author(s) and contributor(s) and not of MDPI and/or the editor(s). MDPI and/or the editor(s) disclaim responsibility for any injury to people or property resulting from any ideas, methods, instructions or products referred to in the content.